Sports Pattern Release

Lorraine Ereira

Sports Pattern Release

Lorraine Ereira

YOUCAXTON PUBLICATIONS
OXFORD & SHREWSBURY

ISBN 978-1-909644-36-6

Printed and bound in Great Britain.

CONTENTS

Part 1
Introduction

Part 2
The Sports Pattern Release Concept

Part 3
Method and Application

FOREWORD

As a founding member of The Society of Sports Therapists, a former lecturer in Sports Science, a Physiotherapist, a coach of elite performers and a qualified and experienced teacher of Physical Education I am always interested to learn of developments or theories around human performance and enhancement. There is much we know about the body but unfortunately more that we do not know; or perhaps it is that we know something about the separate parts but don't understand how the body functions in its most complete sense.

The holistic approach to managing performance and to treating injuries has been an aim that many share but most fail to comprehend because of the complexities of the functions of the body. In this book Lorraine Ereira has evolved and developed her own philosophies based around several aspects of known theories of human function and performance and links several of these strands to form her own unique formulae.

Lorraine discusses the different stages through which the treatment plan progresses and gives examples of when and how to apply each technique. Her own theories are in part drawn from works of other eminent authors which are then used to expand into Lorraine's more encompassing philosophy.

Lorraine may well have pieced together some answers that will take us nearer to a more complete understanding of human performance. Only time, further experimentation and research will determine where Lorraine's work fits in the jigsaw that is human performance.

What is clear is that Lorraine has a desire to find answers and I am sure this book will be just the beginning of that quest. I wish her luck with this book and her continued search for a more comprehensive understanding of human performance.

Keith Waldon MSc. Cert. Ed. MSST MCSP

Sports Pattern Release (SPR) is intended to help manual therapists who work in sport to achieve new and greater results with their patients.

This book will encourage you to build upon your current treatment techniques, develop new hands-on skills and guide your practice to the next level.

By learning the skills involved in Sports Pattern Release, you will discover how to bring about positive changes to your patients' symmetry and alignment, making the way they move both in the sporting context and in everyday life, more balanced and efficient, solving a variety of issues that other treatments may have failed to address.

In this book:

- You will learn the principles of Sports Pattern Release
- You will enhance your knowledge of functional movement
- You will learn a powerful new technique that your patients will want to recommend to others

ACKNOWLEDGEMENTS

Writing this book has been an incredible journey and one that I could have not have done alone.

Firstly, I would like to thank my friend and colleague Ellen Scott for being part of the initial concept development and also for her input into the proof reading of the book.

My thanks also to dear friend and colleague Robyn Burbridge, for her valued input and suggestions.

I would also like to say a thank you to my friend Lesley Hawker, whose interest in this project has both supported and encouraged me to continue.

Huge thanks to Imogen Ereira for her steadfast professional commitment to the formatting and editing of the book.

I would like to thank my photographer Lauren Madgewick for her time and effort in taking and editing the photos for Sports Pattern Release.

Many thanks also to my models Natalie Hawker, for her graceful yoga poses, and my two wonderful sons Jacob and Daniel Ereira, for giving me their time to model for my book.

I would also like to give special thanks to my amazing husband Simeon Ereira, who is always my rock and gives me the confidence in myself to believe I can achieve whatever I put my mind to.

Last, but definitely not least, I need to thank all my patients for allowing me to develop and hone the Sports Pattern Release technique with them, so that I could write this book and bring my concept to other sports therapists.

Lorraine Ereira

PART ONE

Introduction

CHAPTER 1

Why I am passionate about sports therapy

I HAVE BEEN A PRACTICING sports therapist for many years. Prior to gaining my Sports Therapy degree at the University of Kent in 2006, I had spent six years working as a sports massage therapist. People often asked if it was through a love for sport that I became a sports therapist. My fascination came with watching how people moved and functioned. Why did some people bend so easily in one direction but could barely move in another? Why was it that some athletes could run with ease or swim so effortlessly? I understood that people were genetically pre-disposed to certain types of movement. For example, sprinters have more fast twitch muscle fibres and marathon runners have more slow twitch fibres, but this still does not explain why one sprinter looks as though he is flying while another, by comparison, seems to be awkward. He may achieve the same time or distance, but his body did not move as naturally. My interest in dynamic movement and how it varied from person to person was at the heart of my desire to learn more about this exciting subject.

My quest for knowledge has never stopped. I always strive to find ways to be the best sports therapist I can be. This gives me my passion for my job. My philosophy is: the minute you stop wanting more is the beginning of the end of a career.

My career

Whilst I was studying and bringing up my two boys, I was fortunate enough to work in a multi-disciplinary practice. This was a wonderful opportunity as I learnt from other practitioners and shared clinical experiences. It was here that I had the pleasure of working with the well-respected Dr Mike Bundy, who went on to be the sports physician for the England rugby team.

After completing my degree I branched out on my own, setting up my own practice, Optimal Physical Function, where I treat athletes from all sports. I thrive on the diversity my work brings. One thing I quickly realised about my chosen career, however, is that the more you know, the more you realise you don't know! Therefore, I am always looking to enhance and build on the knowledge I have.

I am lucky that my career often consists of contract work, which enables me to expand and develop my skills. This work has included: two seasons working for the GB Lions - Britain's very own American football team; a season working for Harlequins rugby team; working for the Spanish ski team in Hintertux, Austria; and, more recently, I worked at DMRC Headley Court, rehabilitating injured military personnel. All of these experiences continue to enrich my quest for knowledge and my aim is always to bring back new skills, to work with on my own patients.

Sports therapy is still a relatively new profession in the UK and we are still striving to achieve the credibility we deserve. Due to this, I have spent time working alongside my governing body, The Society of Sports Therapists, to try to gain further understanding of how we are moving forward as a profession. This is a personal passion for me. As sports therapists we still have some hurdles to jump, but we are very close to becoming the recognised profession we deserve to be. I would like the Sports Pattern Release (SPR) technique to be another string to add to our already strong bow, giving us that important edge in providing a top service for any athlete.

My testimonials

My reason for writing this book is to share the valuable and interesting experiences that have led me to the development of a technique that will complement and become part of mainstream sports therapy practice.

My clinical career has spanned over some years and I have been fortunate to work with some amazing colleagues and patients. Some of them have kindly written testimonials about my work.

"When Lorraine graduated from the University of Kent in 2006 with a degree in Sports Therapy she joined a growing profession, Sports Therapy, started by The Society of Sports Therapists.

"Lorraine quickly began to explore her professional status and established herself as a leading light in Sports Therapy. She started her own now well-established Sports Injury clinic in Surrey. Lorraine also used the specialist skills in sports trauma management to work pitch-side in a number of sports including Rugby and American Football. Lorraine was one of the first Sports Therapists to work for the GB Lions and started a legacy in American Football in the UK which it is hoped will continue as Sports Therapy assumes its rightful position as the leading profession for pitch-side therapy.

"Lorraine came to my notice when she volunteered her services to work unpaid for The Society of Sports Therapists (the Society). She accompanied me on some of my official duties as a Director of the Society to learn of the work we do so that she could assist us to progress her profession.

"More recently Lorraine was successful in winning the Bruce Hobbs Travelling scholarship and used the funds to work with the Spanish Ski Team during one of their training camps. Lorraine presented her account of the work she did at the Society's AGM in 2011 and, in so doing, became one of the few members to have achieved such status.

"Lorraine continues to campaign for her Society as well as work at her clinic and do a dozen other things in the cause of her profession, one of which is to write this book.

"Lorraine is a remarkable lady and now very much a remarkable Sports Therapist. I wish her well with this book and in her career."

Keith Waldon
Vice Chairman, The Society of Sports Therapists

"I have known Lorraine for many years and have worked with her with many athletes. She is an excellent Sports Therapist who gets great results. I would recommend her to any sports person wanting to see improvement from manual therapy."

Dr Mike Bundy
Senior Team Doctor England RFU 2002-2012, Specialist Sports Physician & Medical Director, Pure Sports Medicine

---

"Lorraine's work with the team had a direct ability on their awareness and physical preparation enabling them to train better when training on skis thereby contributing to their performance.

"The team found her work to be most proficient. She maintained a good balance of familiarity for effective work, with impersonality to remain professional.

"We learnt a lot from Lorraine, particularly in regard to injury prevention."

Mark Tilston
Women's Head Coach, Spanish Alpine Ski Team

"As an elite athlete we have opportunities to work with many excellent therapists and Lorraine was one of them. She helped me with my recovery but she also taught me how to prevent future injuries."

Carolina Ruiz
Spanish Women's Alpine Ski Team

"My physical fitness is very important, and Lorraine's Sports Therapy Treatments are a great support in my preparation for competing on the European Tour."

Peter Fowler
Australian International Golfer

"Always great treatment from Lorraine."

Ceri Jones
Harlequins 2003-2011

"I first had the pleasure of working with Lorraine for the GB Lions American Football Team over five years ago. I found her exceptionably knowledgeable in her clinical work and practical application. She is very approachable and always adheres to the highest of professional standards."

Ellen Scott
England and GB Women's Basketball Sports Therapist

What patients are saying about Sports Pattern Release (SPR)

"I feel so much straighter and more aligned."

Dressage rider

"I've had pelvic and hip pain for years. No-one has been able to get rid of it. After even the first SPR session, I felt much more balanced, and my hip pain was so much better!"

Equestrian

"My legs feel amazing - more energised, more efficient, so much less tired."

Marathon runner

"I was getting constant cramps but since having this treatment, they have gone."

Dressage rider

"Its strange, but the pain in my Achilles' has disappeared, even though that area was not treated at all!"

Marathon runner

"Whatever you did has worked wonders! I didn't even know I had a problem with my gait, but now I feel so much better!"

Walker

I would like to say that all my patients and colleagues have been influential in some way on my journey as a sports therapist and in developing Sports Pattern Release. Without them, I wouldn't be writing this book!

CHAPTER 2

The birth of a concept

SPORTS PATTERN RELEASE HAS its roots in several techniques and concepts, which will be explored throughout this book, but the initial seed was planted in my mind whilst working for the GB Lions, American football team at the Tri-nations Camp in the summer of 2009.

During my time working with the GB Lions, I had the pleasure of working with a colleague, Ellen Scott, for whom I will always have a great respect. The two of us would share ideas and clinical experiences, blending our knowledge and techniques, introducing improved ways to clinically problem solve.

One of the players presented with recurrent hamstring hypertonicity. We treated him in all the conventional ways; massage, soft tissue release, PNF etc., but this issue would return as soon as he trained or competed. He was always on the sidelines being stretched out by one of us because his hamstrings had cramped up again.

After discussing the player's treatment as a team, we finally decided to experiment with a different approach, based on the D1/D2 neuromuscular myofascial patterns, taking the player's lower limb through a fuller range to apply a more universal stretch (see Chapter 3). The next day the player informed us that, although his legs felt a bit tired, they felt much more flexible. This remarkable improvement was seen over the rest of the tournament. We repeated the technique on him and on other players with similar issues and had excellent results all round!

Back in my clinic, I began to apply this technique on some of my athletic patients. It was quite a radical and uncomfortable treatment which left patients tired for about two days. After that, the results were very positive and more athletes came into my clinic asking for the treatment. Very soon I began to form a model, using the treatment two days before an event. This was based on the knowledge that, for optimal results, any inflammatory response triggered by the treatment in the tissues would need 48 hours to recover before training. Patients would text or call me, saying they had performed the best ever, their legs had never felt better - I had 100% success rate!

For two years I sat on this technique, using it on my patients but doing little else with it. However, athletes talk, and before long I had people calling me to ask if they could have "that amazing stretch thing you do".

About a year ago, I began to pursue yoga on a personal level. Before long, I realised that the intense, sustained, diagonal pattern holds, coupled with the diaphragmatic breathing had some similarities to the technique I was using, as my own flexibility and strength took on a new lease of life!

Earlier this year, whilst working at Headley Court, I was introduced to the rolling patterns (which will be discussed in Chapter 3). I also became interested in the fascial sling/network concept. Whilst working there, I realised that yoga was becoming a modality that the military was encouraging. The popularity of yoga in the military is thanks to people like the inspirational Suzie Jennings and her "Heroes at Ease" programme, helping hundreds of injured soldiers. I ensured that all my patients at Headley Court undertook yoga as part of their rehabilitation! They loved it - and they could feel the benefits!

I realised as I continued to practice the Sports Pattern Release technique that it needed some refining, to improve and evolve. With a lot of help from my very willing patients, I worked on it and changed aspects of it until, eventually, I had a technique that I could no longer keep to myself!

All these experiences have led me on my path to Sports Pattern Release - a technique that I hope you will enjoy and, more importantly, for which your patients will reccomend you!

How we typically look at movement dysfunction

A patient presents in the clinic with pain in a specific area. This directs us to ask questions about the localised and notably related tissues and devise a treatment plan. If the injury is acute, then this is the correct course of action. However, sometimes it is a dysfunction of a tissue which is in a chronic state and which does not necessarily fit with localised assessment and treatment protocols.

To illustrate this point let us assume a patient presents with pain in the gluteus maximus region. The role of this large powerful muscle is fairly complex. Primarily its action is to extend and laterally rotate the hip and, while its lower fibres assist in adduction, its upper fibres assist in abduction. Indirectly, as it inserts into the iliotibial band, it helps to stabilise the knee during extension. Additionally, if a patient presents with pain in the gluteus maximus, clinical examination would need to include its innervation from the inferior gluteal nerve as it originates from sacral plexus from the dorsal L5, S1, and S2 rami. Associated tissues that connect with the ileum, sacrum, coccyx and the aponeurosis of the erector spinae, the sacrotuberous ligament and the gluteal aponeurosis may also need to be assessed. Its insertions into the iliotibial band and the gluteal tuberosity of the femur should also be considered. Quite a lot to assess, for just one muscle! However, if we think of dysfunctional tissues in terms of movement and our assessment changes considerably.

Once the related joints and neurological involvement have been assessed, with any pathological factors ruled out, we can think in terms of movement patterning instead of separate structures. The actions of the gluteus maximus, as an individual tissue, takes on less significance. We know from studying the human anatomy that muscles do not work alone. Identifying which individual fibres are most effected, in terms of specific inhibitions or over activity, we also need to look at the bigger picture.

What typical patterns of movements does not only the gluteus maximus, but also its related structures, need to achieve?

For example: Is this patient a runner? How does he need to move? As he extends his hip, he also engages his contra-lateral thoracolumbar fascia connecting the thorax, pelvis and leg, pre-loading through that line during extension to create power in the opposing line as the hip comes through into flexion. However, if this line is weak or restricted in any way, it is going to affect his running gait.

Correcting the overused/tight structures in a directional manner will address the patient's movement, in the direction of treatment, in a way that treating just one structure in one position will not.

PART 2

The Sports Pattern Release Concept

❖

CHAPTER 3

A synergy of methods

Synergy: 'The interaction or co-operation of two or more organizations, substances, or other agents to produce a combined effect greater than the sum of their separate effects.'
New Oxford Dictionary of English

IN THIS CHAPTER WE will review some of the practices and techniques that have given weight to the theory that underpins the Sports Pattern Release (SPR) concept. Many clinicians both treat and rehabilitate patients using these widely-accepted practices. We will discuss each theory and its significance to SPR.

PNF patterns

PNF (proprioceptive neuromuscular facilitation) or, in osteopathic practice, a similar set of principles (muscle energy techniques), was originally used for the rehabilitation of stroke victims. These techniques were first developed by Herman Kabat[1] a neurophysiologist who used the principles of neuromuscular facilitation and inhibition in natural movements. In the 1950s, assisted by Dorothy Voss and Margaret Knott[2], he began to teach and present the technique. Universities teaching physical therapy in the 1960s began to include this in their courses. This utilised what we know about agonist and antagonistic behaviour and the fact that the body works in different directions at the same time.

His methods are still used today in clinical practice and still have great effects.

However the most significant part of Kabat's methods, and the methods of other clinicians who have successfully used these techniques, is that he believed that combinations of movement were more beneficial than moving one joint at a time. The application of the PNF patterns will be explained in Chapter 5.

Rolling patterns

Gray Cook's rolling patterns also bear relevance to the SPR technique as they require length throughout the diagonal and rotational movements of the body. Cook refers to the fact that when we enter this world we are fully functionally mobile. Babies are able to roll, crawl and squat by instinct, they do not have to be taught these movements and, in fact, as we grow up we unlearn them! When we, as infants, learn to stabilise we do so reflexively, from the trunk, in order to control more distal movement. It is only later in life, due to poor training, injuries or during the activities of daily living, that we develop compensatory movements that lead to asymmetries in the body.

Rolling patterns combine the use of the upper extremities, the core and the lower extremities in a co-ordinated manner to get from one position to another - a movement that, although primitive in its essence, requires tissue length and proper sequencing of the body segments in order to reflexively stabilise and make the move effectively.

The flexibility factor is critical here - i.e. this cannot be executed and taught as a stability exercise if there is insufficient mobility in the tissues. If there is insufficient length or restrictions during sling activation/strength training, then the mechanics of the exercise become compromised. Thus if the patient does not have the mobility to achieve these starting patterns pain free, then the patient will just learn compensatory movements and the exercise becomes pointless. By contrast, if the patient is hypermobile and too easily able to get to into the position prior to executing the roll, he will not have the strength required to complete the roll and therefore will need to strengthen that particular movement pattern. A good understanding of this is necessary in order to learn this technique and to be able teach it to patients.

Once there is enough mobility to disassociate the pelvis from the shoulder girdle, then the inner core muscles can be engaged (transversus abdominus, multifidus, diaphragm and pelvic floor, prior to obliques, rectus abdominis and quadratus lumborum). It can be done from prone to supine and supine to prone, with either arm or leg leading, either way. This is especially beneficial for any athlete involved in rotational based sport (golf, throwing, tennis, swimming, dance, gymnastics, to name a few) but can also help to identify weakness or over activity in any individual.

Based on the PNF principles, the rolling patterns can be used to treat and train patients both with neurological dysfunction and musculoskeletal conditions. They utilise the PNF principles of irradiation or overflow. In simple terms, by facilitating the stronger portion of a pattern, the motor unit activation of the weaker portion is enhanced, strengthening the response of the involved segments.

Below are the four rolling pattern movements as summarised from an article in the North American Journal of Sports Physical Therapy.[3]

In Figure 3.1 , the first pattern is described in detail with the cues. The following figures only describe the pattern as the cues and principles are the same.

Fig 3.1: Supine to prone - arm leading

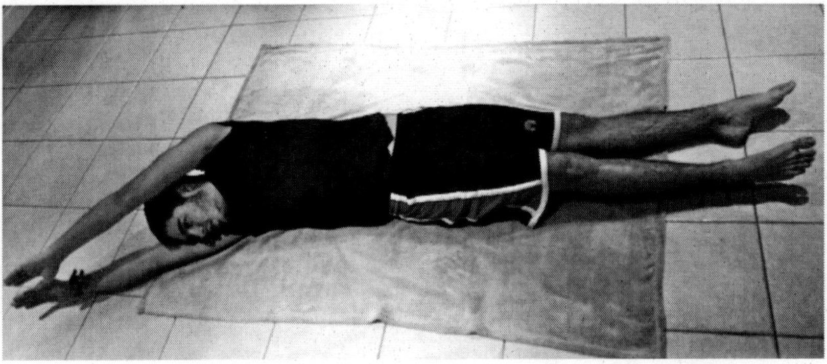

This pattern begins with shoulder flexion/adduction, leading to trunk flexion/rotation and ending in pelvic rotation/hip flexion.

The move is begun by laying supine with arms in full flexion and legs in full extension.

The patient is asked to roll in the above sequence. The patient's head and neck should flex and the trunk rotates towards the axilla of the direction they are rolling in, (i.e. to the right, in the example above). The lower body should not contribute to the roll. The patient should be instructed to focus on length, i.e. lengthening the left leg and the right arm. The patient can be cued to push his opposite shoulder into the floor to act as a driver. Only when his shoulders are perpendicular to the floor (i.e. stacked) should his hip leave the floor to complete the rotation.

Fig 3.2: Prone to supine - arm leading

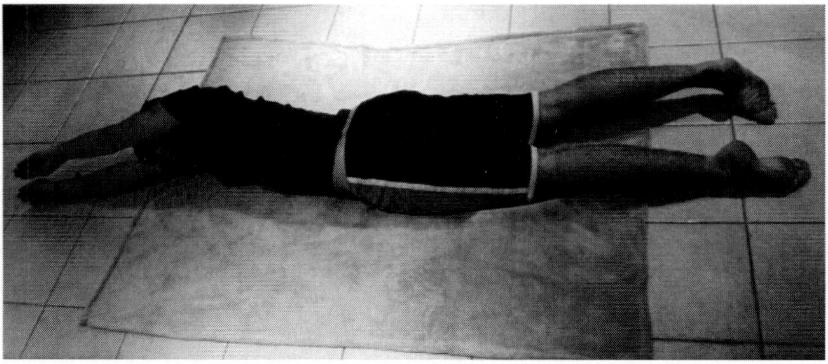

This pattern begins with shoulder flexion, then trunk extension/rotation and finishes with pelvic rotation.

Fig 3.3: Supine to prone - leg leading

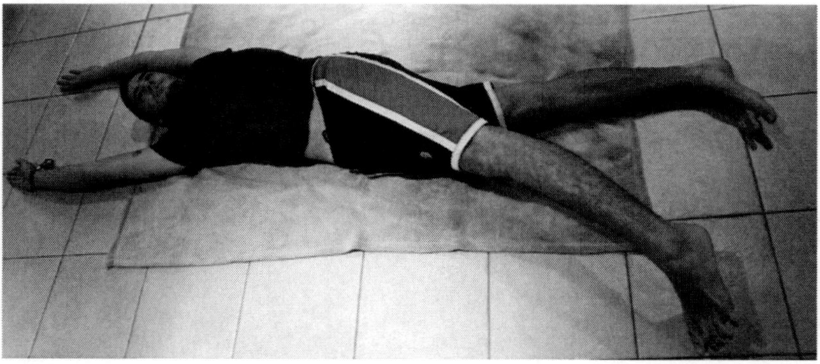

This pattern begins with hip flexion, leading to pelvic rotation/lumbar flexion and finishes with trunk flex and rotation.

Once again, the patient needs to lengthen the unmoving leg and can drive with the same hip. He must not lift the opposite shoulder until his hip girdle is perpendicular to the floor.

Fig 3.4: Prone to supine - leg leading

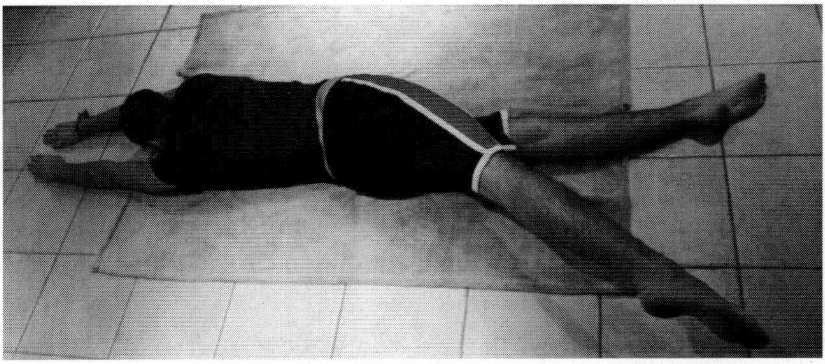

Beginning with hip extension, leading to pelvic rotation and lumbar extension. Finishing with trunk extension and rotation.

The rolling patterns have influenced Sports Pattern Release because they work with diagonal and rotational movement patterns. The principles of symmetry and balance throughout the body are recognised as fundamental to injury prevention and correction of dysfunction.

Yoga and breathing

Training the body for any sport has for many years focused on muscle strength, cardiovascular conditioning and neuromuscular co-ordination - all of which are of great importance. Current thinking takes us back to the timeless practice of yoga, which has always focused on movement patterns, both strengthening and lengthening the body, not as individual parts, but as whole sequences of poses that develop the function of the body in an unrivaled way.

The other key focus of yogic practice is breathing, something that is all too often overlooked but is of the utmost importance in correct biomechanical function. The human body will sacrifice everything to maintain respiratory function and this includes posture. Nasal breathing is the way we are pre-programmed to breathe and mouth breathing is triggered by stress. Interestingly, when posture is poor, it is easier to breathe through the mouth and harder to breathe nasally. The reverse is also true, illustrating the close relationship between breathing and posture. Additionally, mouth breathers often breathe much less deeply, only using the upper chest, whereas nose breathers tend to use the diaphragm making full use of the lungs, oxygenating the blood and brain. If the diaphragm becomes inhibited through poor posture, stress or bad habits, the accessory inhibitory muscles will overwork, becoming overactive, leading to trigger points and chronic tension.

There are many different yoga breathing exercises. Pranayama breathing, which is the practice of voluntary breath control, when practised slowly has been shown to have positive effects on immune function, hypertension, asthma, autonomic nervous system imbalances and psychological or stress-related disorders. Jerath, R. *et al.*, 2006, hypothesised that voluntary slow deep breathing functionally resets the autonomic nervous system.[4] Investigations have demonstrated that slow pranayama breathing techniques activate the parasympathetic (inhibitory) nervous system. This type of breathing employed with deep stretching will have a combined effect on stimulating parasympathetic activity while concurrently decreasing sympathetic activity. This will lower the heart rate, blood pressure and induce relaxation.

Breathing diaphragmatically during SPR is critical to the treatment. This is because, if the patient is not coached to use this type of breathing, he may find the somewhat intense positions and the palpation of tender myofascial points, uncomfortable. The anxiety of being taken into potentially uncomfortable ranges, coupled with the pre-tensing of tissue in anticipation of possible pain, stimulates the production of adrenalin. This in turn triggers the sympathetic nervous response which can make the patient feel hot, nauseous and lightheaded during the treatment. Therefore, diaphragmatic breathing is crucial to the successful administration and results of the SPR method.

Yoga based exercise and correct breathing education can provide an excellent follow-up to the SPR technique, if the exercises are given with the appropriate professional understanding of how they support the clinical application. This will be discussed further in Chapter 9.

Trigger points

The term "trigger point" was coined by Dr Janet Travell in 1942. The trigger point model, or hyper-irritable muscle knots, are local points in the skeletal muscles that refer pain to remote locations in the body. The trigger point concept bears relevance to Sports Pattern Release because the main foundation of Travell's theory is based on myofascial pain – the combination of muscle and fascia.[5] The trigger point is formed as a knot of locally contracted muscle fibres, which then pull on tendons and joints associated with that muscle, causing pain. The sustained contraction of these fibres compress the local blood supply, restricting the energy to that region. This lack of energy produces substances which irritate the nociceptive or pain nerves which then produce pain within muscle tissue at the neuromuscular junction.[6] There will often be weakness in the associated structures as they have a poor blood supply and poor neural pathways.

It has been documented that trigger pointing works more effectively if used in conjunction with stretching techniques.[7] An important aspect of SPR is the stretching which is applied at the end of each stage of the treatment. The timing and application of the stretch is also a key factor.

The trigger points

Fig 3.5: Anterior view

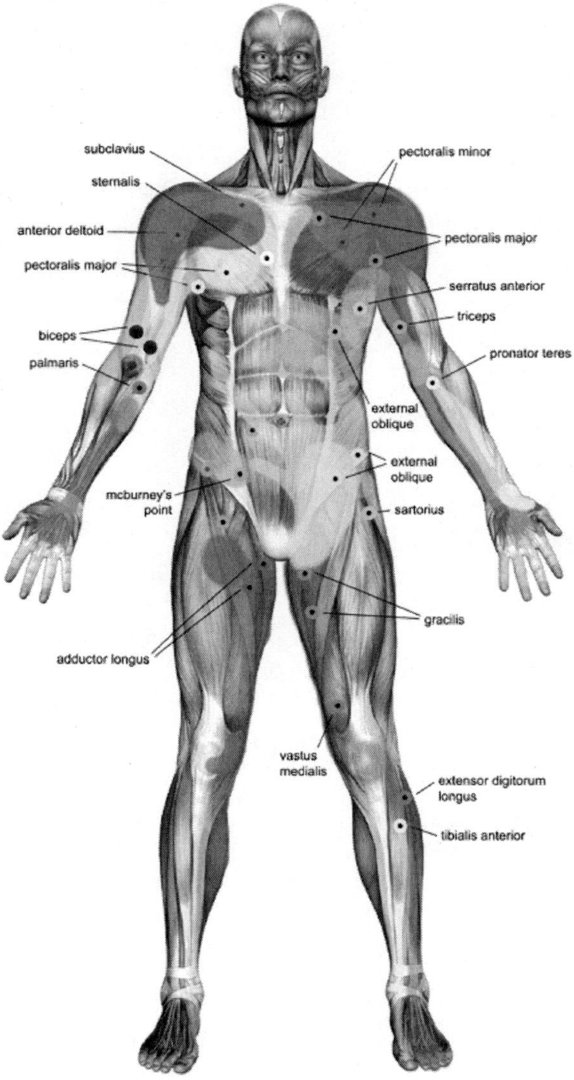

Reprinted with permission of Trigger Point Performance® the leader in Performance Therapy. www.tptherapy.com

Fig 3.6: Posterior view

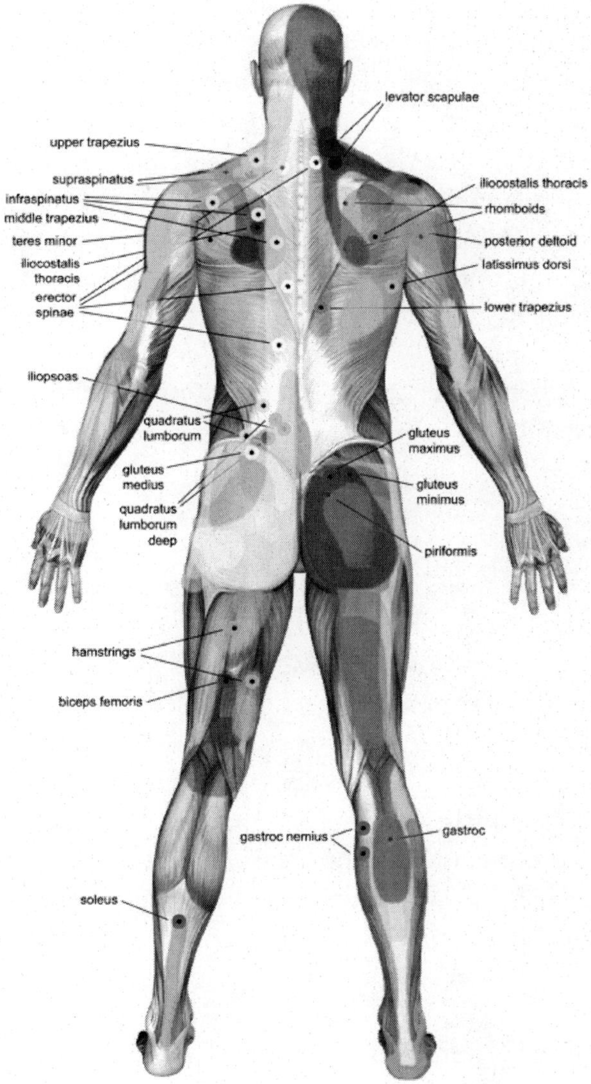

Reprinted with permission of Trigger Point Performance® the leader in Performance Therapy. www.tptherapy.com

Joints

One area that is rarely covered when we think in terms of functional movement treatment is the accessory movement of the joints. The majority of techniques, discussed earlier in this book and indeed by other clinicians, focus almost solely on the soft tissues. As stated earlier, focusing on any one structure to the exclusion of others is impractical, as every moving part has an influence on another moving part. Joints are also a key consideration when thinking of integrated or connected movement.

It is a vital part of the SPR technique to consider joint restrictions; perhaps it is this element that sets it apart from many other treatment procedures. If it is not within the reader's scope of practice to treat the joints, the patient should be referred to the relevant professional. However, if the soft tissue part of the technique is utilised, the effects are still hugely beneficial. This aspect of the technique will be discussed further in Chapter 7.

Neural tension

Just as joint or soft tissue restrictions can occur and cause symptoms in the body, restrictions of the nervous systems mechanics can also cause pain. Some of the sports patterns will place the patient in a position of neural tension, which can sometimes induce either presenting symptoms or other symptoms, such as pins and needles or numbness. Neural tension can be secondary to soft tissue lesions or due to primary damage to neural tissue. Neural mobilisation may be an effective method of restoring normal neural mechanics by the restoration of the dynamic balance between the relative movement of neural tissues and surrounding mechanical boundaries, thereby allowing a reduction in intrinsic pressures on the neural tissue and thus promoting optimum physiologic function.[8]

However, it should be noted that care must be taken in acute or irritable conditions as these stretches may aggravate the symptoms. If neural symptoms do arise during the SPR treatment, it should only be continued if the clinician is suitably qualified and experienced to deal with neurological conditions.

References

(1) Sharman, M., Cresswell, A., and Reik S. (2006). PNF stretching. *sports medicine.* 36 (1), p.929-939.

(2) McTee, R.E., Charland, J (1999). *Facilitated Stretching.* Champaign (IL): Human Kinetics. P.14

(3) Hoogenboom, B.J., Voight, M.J., Cook, G., Gill, L. (2009). Using Rolling to Develop Neuromuscular Control and Coordination of the Core and Extremities of Athletes. *N Am J Sports Physical Therapy. May.* 4 (2), p.70-82.

(4) Jerath,R., Edry, J.W., Barnes, V.A., Jerath, V. (2006). Physiology of long pranayamic breathing: Neural respiratory elements may provide a mechanism that explains how slow deep breathing shifts the autonomic nervous system. *Epub.* 67 (3), p.566-71.

(5) Jantos, M. (2007). Understanding Chronic Pelvic Pain. *Pelvipherineology.* 26 (2)

(6) Travell, J., Simons, D., Simons, L. (1999). *Myofascial Pain and Dysfunction: The Trigger Point Manual.* 2nd ed. USA: Lippincott Williams & Williams.

(7) Lewit, K., Simons, D.G. (1984). Myofascial pain: Relief by post-isometric relaxation. *Archives of Physical Medicine and Rehabilitation.* 65 (8), p.452-6.

(8) Ellis, R.F., Hing, W.A. (2008). Neural Mobilisation: A Systematic Review of Randomized Controlled Trials with an Analysis of Therapeutic Efficacy. *Journal of Manual & Manipulative Therapy.* 16 (1), p.8-22.

CHAPTER 4

Slings: both fascial and functional

A MAJOR INFLUENCE IN THE Sports Pattern Release (SPR) technique is the role and function of slings. This subject is exemplified in Tom Myers' *Anatomy Trains*, where he brings us the principles of myofascial meridians. Myers describes the myofascial meridians as the *"Lines of pull which transmit strain and movement round the bodies myofascia round the skeleton."* (Myers, T. 2009). He cites Schultz and Feitis in his book, who summarise the role of connective tissue thus: *"The muscle-bone concept presented in standard anatomical description gives a purely mechanical mode of movement. It separates movement into discrete functions, failing to give a picture of the seamless integration seen in a living body. When one part moves the body as a whole responds. Functionally the only tissue in the body that can mediate such responsiveness is connective tissue.*[9] *"*

Myers outlines the way fascia works in one word, "tensegrity". This is simply the relationship between tension and compression. It is explained as a single force in one part of the body, having an effect throughout the body. The fascia creates the structure around the contracting and relaxing muscles.

Anatomy Trains illustrates these forces in specific lines throughout the body. These lines are engaged during movement but primarily in postural control.

There are marked similarities between Myers' *Anatomy Trains* and Andry Vleeming's postural slings. The key difference is that postural slings do not span the entire body, whereas myosfascial slings can run from head to toe. This means that it would be unlikely for a whole myofascial sling to be engaged during a particular movement, whereas postural slings are activated in their entirety. Myofascial slings can be anatomically connected without being functionally related and so restrictions in the myofascial chain are more likely to be localised. However, it has been shown that releasing areas of myofascia can help with postural dysfunctions. For example, releasing a restriction in the plantar fascia, a component of the superficial back line, can improve the ability to forward bend to touch the toes. Yet for dynamic or motor dysfunction, the postural slings may have more clinical relevance.[10]

The postural slings are described as the muscular systems dynamic way to stabilise joints. The principles of particular lines of force again apply here, but Vleeming's postural or myofascial slings were mainly focused on force closure (the compression of opposing forces in the soft tissue, ligaments and fascia), particularly around the sacro-iliac joint, giving it stability when form closure (the congruency of the articulating joint surfaces) was not able to provide the correct level of stabilisation for healthy function. The hypothesis is that the postural slings have no beginning or end. The parts of the slings identified below are relative to a particular movement pattern or motion which has been activated during that pattern.

It has been noted that athletes who are involved in high impact sport often experience dysfunction of these slings, due to overload of the pelvic ligaments and sacro-iliac joint.

Postural slings are divided into four main groups:

- The anterior oblique sling
- The posterior oblique sling
- The deep longitudinal sling
- The lateral sling

Fig 4.1: The anterior oblique sling

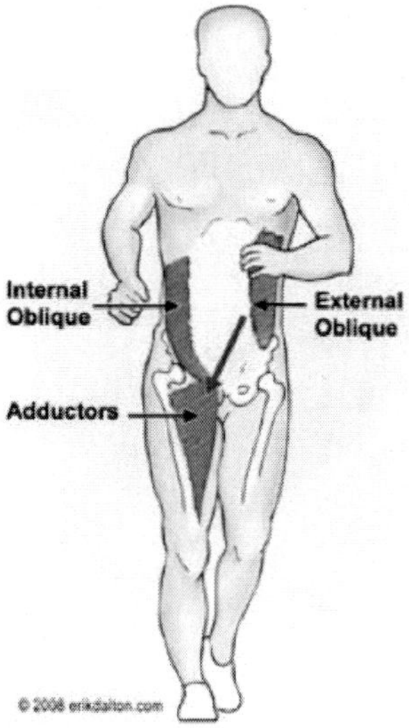

Pectorals

Contralateral adductors

Obliques (internal and external)

Abdominal fascia

Reproduced with permission from Erik Dalton, Ph.D

Fig. 4.2: The posterior oblique sling

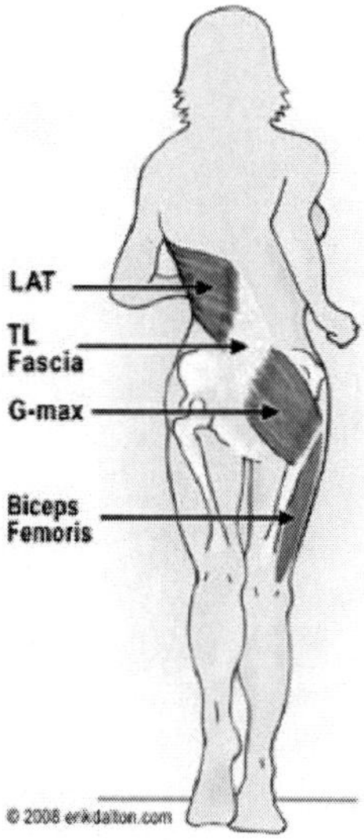

Latissimus dorsi

Contralateral glut max and biceps femoris

Reproduced with permission from Erik Dalton, Ph.D

Fig 4.3: The deep longitudinal sling

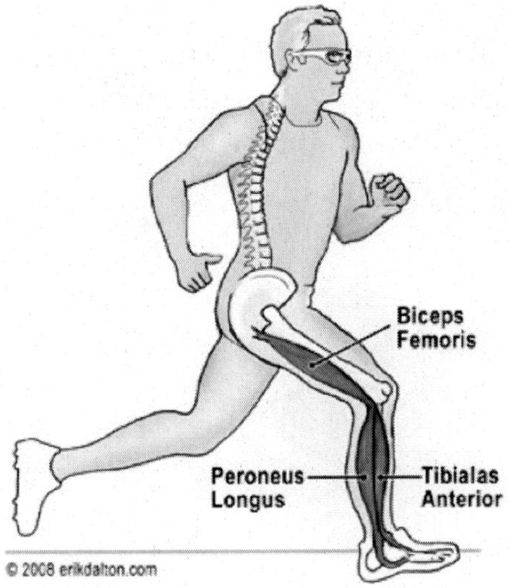

Erector spinae and spinal fascia

Deep layer of thoracolumbar fascia

The sacrotuberous ligament via the longhead of biceps femoris and peroneus longus

Reproduced with permission from Erik Dalton, Ph.D

Fig 4.4: The lateral sling

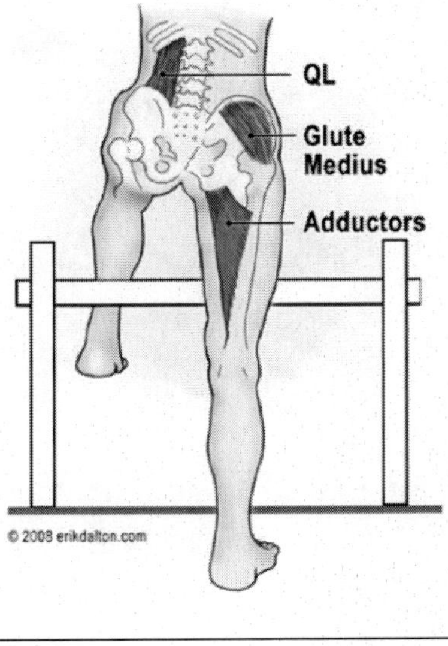

Gluteus medius and minimus

Ipsilateral adductors

Contralateral quadratus lumborum

Reproduced with permission from Erik Dalton, Ph.D

The anterior oblique sling (Figure 4.1) works to compress the abdominal contents, compressing the pelvic girdle and stabilising the symphysis pubis. The adductors work in harmony with the internal oblique and contralateral external oblique to both stabilise the body on the same stance leg and rotate the pelvis forward. This sling is perhaps the most relevant in multi-directional sport, as it contributes to acceleration, deceleration and changing direction. This can be exemplified by any patient who has had an abdominal or groin strain, as these movements will cause immediate pain.

The posterior oblique sling (Figure 4.2) provides stability to the sacro-iliac joint by acting on the sacrotuberous ligaments and the thoracolumbar fascia. As the latissimus dorsi and contralateral gluteus maximus co-contract, tension is produced in the thoracolumbar fascia helping to stabilise the sacro-iliac joint of the stance leg.

The deep longitudinal sling (Fig 4.3) also works to stabilise the pelvis and the sacro-iliac joint by contraction of the multifidus and the thoracolumbar fascia. The spinal erectors communicate with the biceps femoris via the sacrotuberous ligament and to the lower limb through the peroneus longus.

The lateral sling (Fig 4.4) provides stability, in the frontal plane, through the co-contraction of the gluteus medius and adductors with the contralateral quadratus lumborum. Weakness or fatigue in this sling can cause excessive stress on ligaments and discs in the pelvis and spine.

Myers agrees that the similarities are indeed present and draws parallels between the anterior and posterior oblique sling and the functional lines, the deep longitudinal and the superficial back line.[11] Yet he purports that the myofascial meridians of the *Anatomy Trains* concept are more focused on fascial connections, whereas other prior concepts are based on functional connections. Both these clinicians undoubtedly recognised the importance of connected tissues and their role in how the body moves.

Is fascia really capable of being influenced by manual therapy?

'Fascia' is a web like tissue that connects a variety of structures in the body. Myofascia is tougher and deeper than the fascial layer which lies beneath the skin. It is a clear, fibrous layer that surrounds muscle tissue. It lies just outside the muscle's epimysium and it binds individual muscles into functional groups via its continuous interconnections with tendons and ligaments.

The study of fascia has become fashionable of late. Although it is important, for any sports therapist or manual therapist to understand the lines of fascia, as they should the different muscles or joints in the body, it is not good to get fixated upon any one structure of the body as the focal point of treatment. We must remember that we exist as complex beings whose anatomical structures are highly dependent on each other to produce movement, maintain posture and indeed to function on any level. Hence, if there is a limitation in one muscle which works in conjunction with another muscle that is bound by the same fascial net to perform a particular movement, and it is also innervated by the same neural pathway, then treating that restriction will help to facilitate that whole movement pattern.

Tom Myers approach, in his book *Anatomy Trains*, recognises and embraces the more global approach to treatment and movement. He states in his book that; *"the body distributes strain, especially chronic strain, in an attempt to equalise the forces on the tissues, and that releasing one area of the body can produce changes some distance away from the intervention."* This theory is well supported by trigger point therapy.

Some clinicians disagree. Chaudhry *et al*, 2008, stated that *"You cannot change the structure of fascia, because it is tougher than Kevlar".* [12] They argue that that fascia itself, although containing a few muscle fibres, has very limited contractile properties, nowhere near as much as muscle tissue. It is commonly thought that the properties of fascia are more viscoelastic or plastic (like a plastic bag) instead of elastic (like an elastic band).

Although fascial contractions may be weak compared to muscles, they could be **powerful** in another way - their effects might, for instance, accumulate over time to produce tissues contractures. So it is still worth considering how these contractions might be clinically relevant.

Understanding stretching: the muscle's stretch reflex

The myotatic stretch reflex's main purpose is to prevent a muscle from stretching too far and thereby prevent injury. One of the reasons for holding a stretch for a prolonged period of time is that, as you hold the muscle in a stretched position, the muscle spindle becomes accustomed to the new length and reduces its signaling. The myotatic reflex stimulates muscular contraction; when muscle is stretched, the muscle spindles also stretch and send sensory impulses to the spinal cord informing the central nervous system that the muscle is being stretched. Impulses then return to that muscle causing the muscle to contract, therefore resisting the stretch. If the stretch is maintained over at least 6-60 secs,[13] the Golgi tendon organ overrides the impulses coming from the muscle spindles causing the muscle to relax, after the initial resistance, to the new length. For this reason, the lengthening and holding method is unlikely to cause any injury to the tissues.

Although the contractile properties of fascia are very different from that of muscle, it also has a very rich mechanoreceptor innervation. Golgi tendon organs work by giving afferent feedback to the spinal cord, causing the motor neurons to reduce their firing rate and thereby decreasing tension in muscle fibre. They also require active muscular contractions to be stimulated. According to Schleip, R. 2003, it is another type of mechanoreceptor that we should be studying, when it comes to fascia.[14] Ruffini corpuscles respond to a stretch that is applied in the same plane as the tissue beneath the pressure being applied. They respond to slow changes in pressure, applied in the line of treatment.

Schleip, R. cites Myers, T., 1997, to sum up part of this process; *"The long myofascial chains are the preferred focus when doing slow dynamic stretches. Instead of stretching isolated muscle groups, the aim is finding body movements that engage the longest possible myofascial chains.*

Multidirectional movements, with slight changes in angle are utilised; this might include sideways or diagonal movement variations as well as spiraling rotations. With this method, large areas of the fascial network are simultaneously involved. By changing the angle slightly, different aspects of the fascial web are addressed with slow and steady movements." [15]

Sports Pattern Release focuses primarily on the postural slings and the back and front functional lines (see Figures 4.5 and 4.6), which are the most relevant for athletic performance and treatment, and secondarily the lateral and spiral lines, as these are the lines that give us power and precision for our movement by lengthening the lever limb and linking it across the body. The arm lines will also have some clinical relevance to the technique as they are extensions to the functional lines.

Fig 4.5: Back functional line

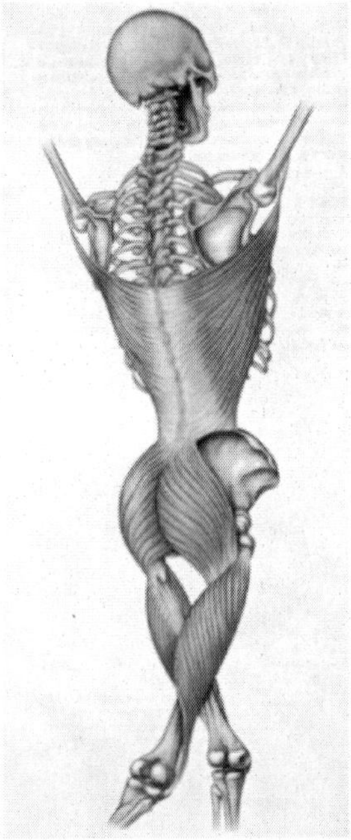

Fig 4.6: Front functional line

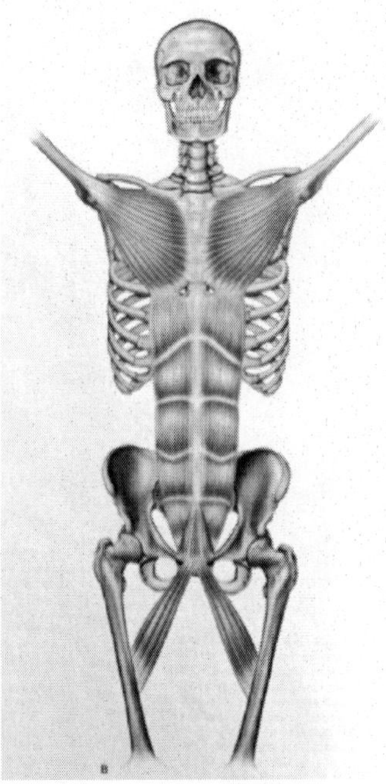

References

(9) Schultz, L., Feitis, R. (1996). *The Endless Web.* Berkeley: North Atlantic Books.

(10) Wadsworth, D. (2007). *Locomotor Slings: A New Total Body Therapists Approach to Treating Chronic Pain.* Available: http://membership.aamt.com.au/lib/Journals/Winter07/Win07-Locomotor.pdf. Last accessed sept 2013.

(11) Myers, T. W. (2009). *Anatomy Trains: Myofascial Meridians for Manual and Movement Therapists.* 2nd ed. London: Churchill Livingstone.

(12) Ingraham, P. (2011). *Three- dimensional mathematical model for deformation of human fasciae in manual therapy.* Available: http://saveyourself.ca/bibliography.php?chaudhry08. Last accessed Nov 2013.

(13) Prentice, W.E (2004). *Rehabilitation Techniques for Sports Medicine and Athletic Training.* 4th ed. Columbus: McGraw-Hill.

(14) Schleip, R. (2003). Fascial plasticity – a new neurobiological explanation: part 1. *Journal of Bodywork and Movement Therapies.* 7, (Issue 1), p11-19.

(15) Schleip, R., D.G. Muller. (2012). Training Principles for Fascial Connective Tissues: Scientific Foundation and Suggested Practical Applications. *Journal of Bodywork & Movement Therapies.* xx, 1-13.

PART 3

Method and Application

CHAPTER 5

Functional patterns for sports and everyday activity

MOST PRACTITIONERS WHO HAVE patients and clients who are athletes also have those who are not. Sports Pattern Release can be applied to any dysfunctional movement and therefore can also help to treat tissue dysfunction that has not been induced by sport.

The more complex activation of the functional lines and postural slings are often preceded by the simple diagonal pattern movements discussed in Chapter 3.

The PNF patterns application

There are eight main patterns for the limbs, four for the upper limbs and four for the lower:

1. Flexion/extension
2. Diagonal: motion towards and across the midline, or across and away from the midline (adduction/abduction)
3. Rotation (internal/external)

These patterns utilise gross movements as opposed to specific muscle actions. They are mimicked in most sports and daily activities. They are functional.

D1 arm pattern
Moving from flexion into extension (grab and fasten seatbelt)

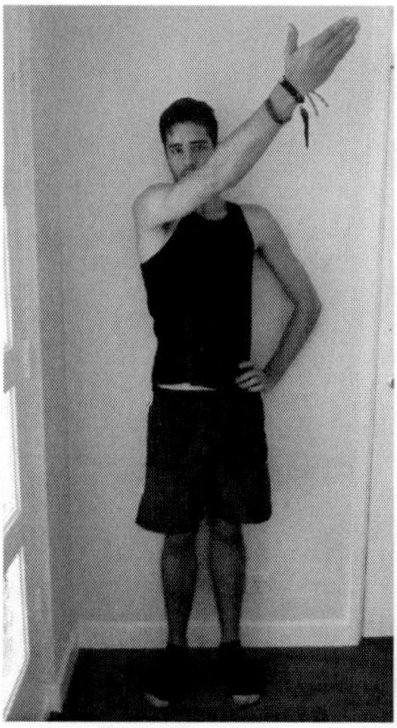

Fig 5.1: Flex-add-ER (D1 flex)

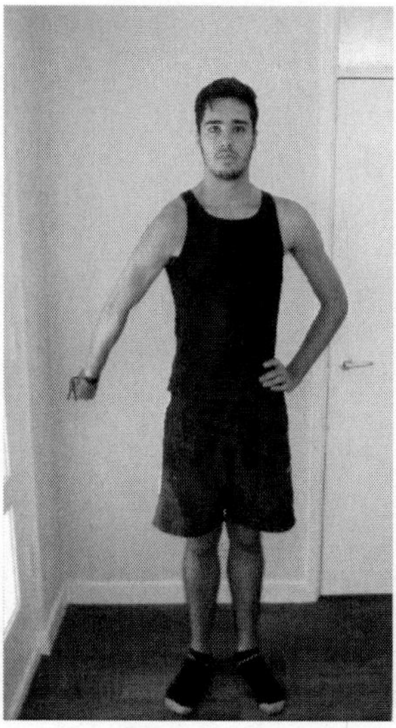

Fig 5.2: Ext-abd-IR (D1 ext)

D2 arm pattern
Moving from extension into flexion (drawing a sword)

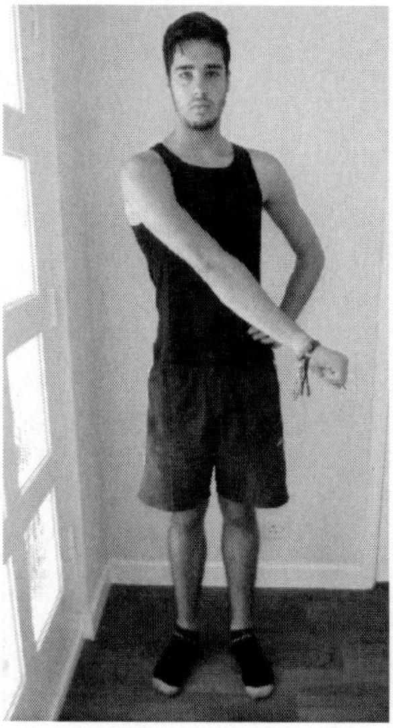

Fig 5.3: Ext-add-IR (D2 ext)

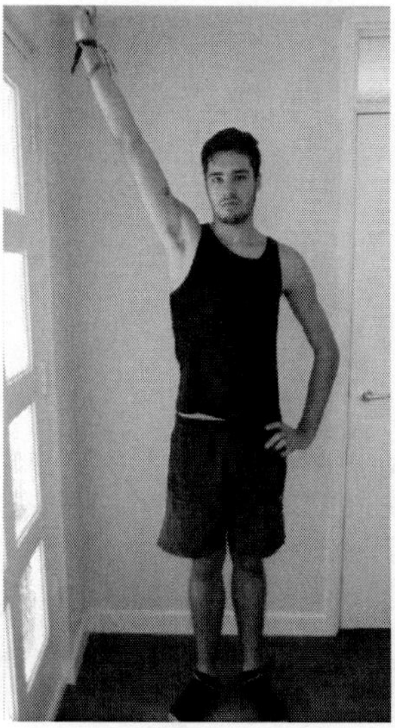

Fig 5.4: Flex-abd-ER (D2 flex)

D1 leg pattern
Moving from flexion into extension (soccer kick)

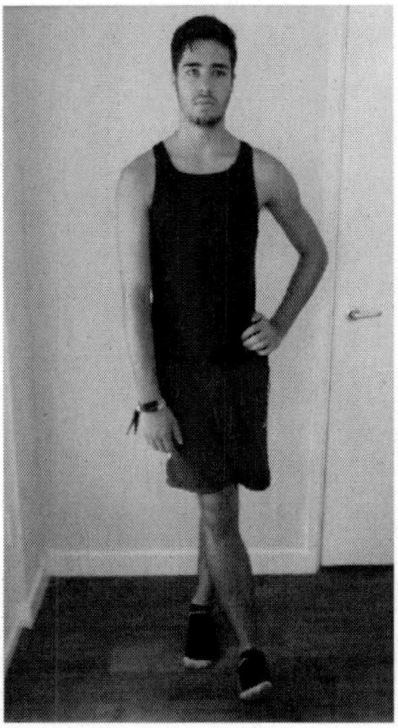
Fig 5.5: Flex-add-ER (D1 flex)

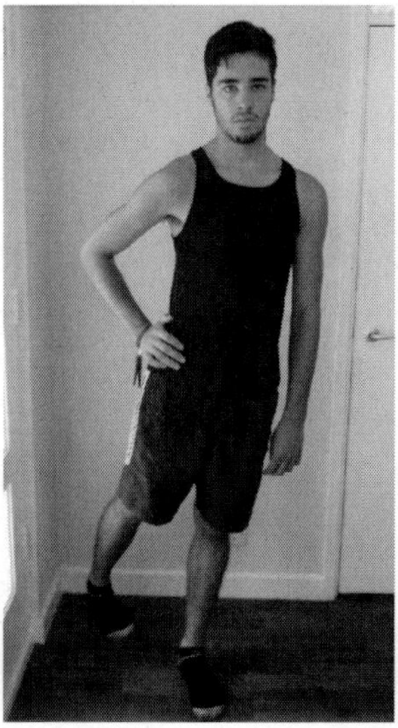
Fig 5.6: Ext-abd-IR (D1 Ext)

D2 leg pattern
Moving from D2 flexion into D2 extension (snow plough/fifth position)

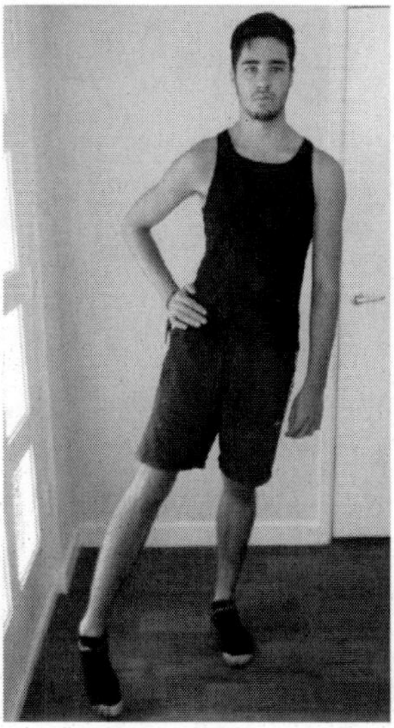
Fig 5.7: Flex-abd-IR (D2 flex)

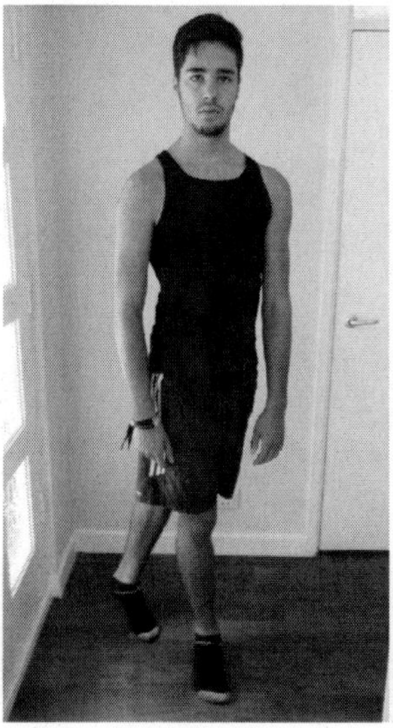
Fig 5.8: Ext-add-ER (D2 Ext)

The patterns are the basis of normal functional movement. Patients often present in clinic with pain or stiffness in a particular region of the body. Although therapists would prefer patients to be very specific as to which movement causes this pain/restriction, the patient can often not tell us. We ask questions like "does it hurt to bend forward/flex to the side/rotate to the left etc.?" but patients do not think like this and, more importantly, they do not move like this, which is why we invariably do not get the required response. What they are more likely to say is "it feels difficult to remove my jacket/get up from sitting/put on my socks etc.". This is a movement pattern, something they can identify with and which can actually tell the therapist much more about their dysfunction! This approach directs our clinical reasoning away from the individual body part and towards functional movement patterning.

Example 1

A patient reports in his subjective examination that he finds it difficult to reach his seatbelt in the car. The beginning of this movement pattern employs a combination of shoulder flexion, adduction and external rotation, moving into internal rotation as he completes the reach. This is the classic D1 PNF flexion pattern pictured in Figure 5.1.

As the patient continues to reach even further into the pattern he begins to rotate the spine from lumbar to cervical. He requires enough length and no restrictions in the superficial back arm line and the back functional line.

The fundamental difference here between an activity of daily living (ADL) and a sports-related movement, is that most ADLs do not require explosive movement in the opposite pattern. This is explained further in Chapter 6.

Example 2

A rugby player presents with stiffness in his spine when kicking a ball. (See Figure 8.3) He needs a good range of movement in his hips (D1 flexion) but, as he rotates his trunk to complete the movement, he also needs to have the flexibility in his lumber spine and also in his opposite shoulder. (See Figure 8.8)

Fig 5.9: Harlequins rugby player being treated in SPR 1 Add Range (lower limb)

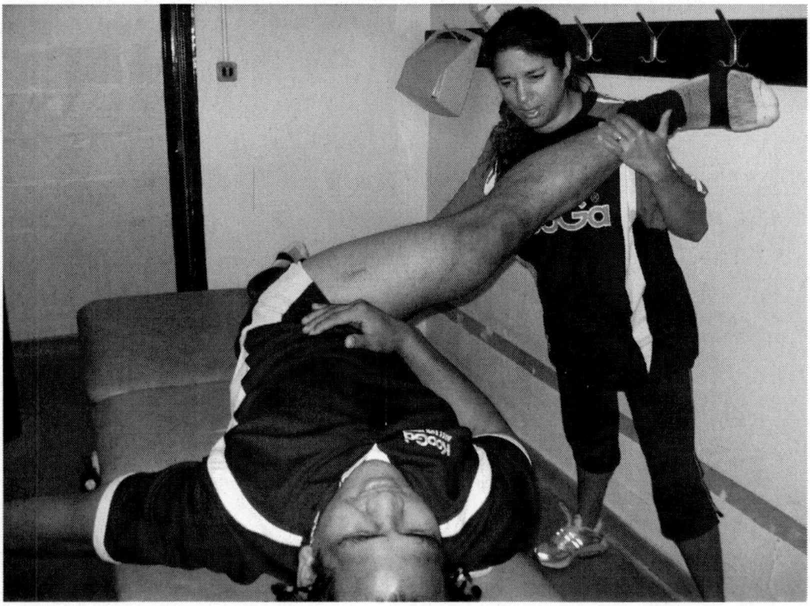

CHAPTER 6

Common sports patterns

THE FUNCTIONAL LINES ARE the ones we associate mostly with the majority of sports-related movement and have a role to play in terms of stabilising the body. Stabilisation is particularly needed during movement, when the body is required to transmit forces from the lower limb to the upper limb.

If you watch an athlete in motion you will notice that these functional lines or slings are almost always engaged in a continuum with each other. For example, the counterbalancing weight of the arms is necessary for the momentum of a kick and the pelvis needs to move to accommodate and give power to a tennis serve. This is easily demonstrated during the simple act of walking. If the arms are held stationary during the gait, it makes walking harder and if the arm swing is opened up, the gait will also increase.

Comparing the anatomy of functional lines to the oblique slings

The back functional line begins with the latissimus dorsi's insertion to the intertubercular groove of the humerous, through the lumbodorsal fascia, joining the sacral fascia. Here it crosses the midline at the sacrolumbar junction to the contralateral lower gluteus maximus fibres. It then passes beneath the iliotibial band to attach to the postero-lateral edge of the femur. It continues through the vastus lateralis through the patella tendon to the tibial tuberosity (Figure 4.5). This follows a very similar track to the to the posterior oblique sling which runs from the latissimus dorsi to the contralateral gluteus maximus and biceps femoris (Figure 4.2).

The front functional line begins on the humeral shaft as well, with the pectoralis major passing along its lower fibres to the fifth and sixth ribs. These lower pectoralis major fibres link into the lateral sheath of the rectus abdominis. Passing through the pubic bone and symphasis, it crosses the body here to the contralateral adductor longus, going down and out to the linea aspera on the posterior femur (Figure 4.6). Once more, it is important to stress its similarity to the anterior oblique sling, which connects the pectorals to the contralateral adductors via the obliques (internal and external) and abdominal fascia (Figure 4.1). Table 6.1 and 6.2 show how closely the functional lines run to the oblique slings.

Table 6.1: Back functional line and posterior oblique sling

	BACK FUNCTIONAL LINE		POSTERIOR OBLIQUE
Orientation	**Bony stations**	**Myofascial tracks**	**Sling connections**
Ipsilateral	1. Shaft of humerus		
		2. Latissimus dorsi	1. Latissimus dorsi
		3. Lumbodorsal fascia	
Contralateral		4. Sacral fascia	
	5. Sacrum		
		6. Gluteus maximus	2. Gluteus maximus
	7. Shaft of femur		
		8. Vastus lateralis	3. Biceps femoris
	9. Patella		
		10. Subpatellar tendon	
	11. Tuberosity of tibia		

Table 6.2: Front functional line and anterior oblique sling

	FRONT FUNCTIONAL LINE		ANTERIOR OBLIQUE
Orientation	**Bony stations**	**Myofascial tracks**	**Sling connections**
Ipsilateral	1. Shaft of humerus		
		2. Lower edge of pectoralis major	1. Pectoralis major
	3. Fifth rib and sixth rib cartilage		
		4. Lateral sheath of rectus abdominis	2. Obliques and abdominal fascia
	5. Pubic tubercle		
Contralateral		6. Adductor longus	3. Adductors
	7. Linea aspera of femur		

Fig 6.1: Running

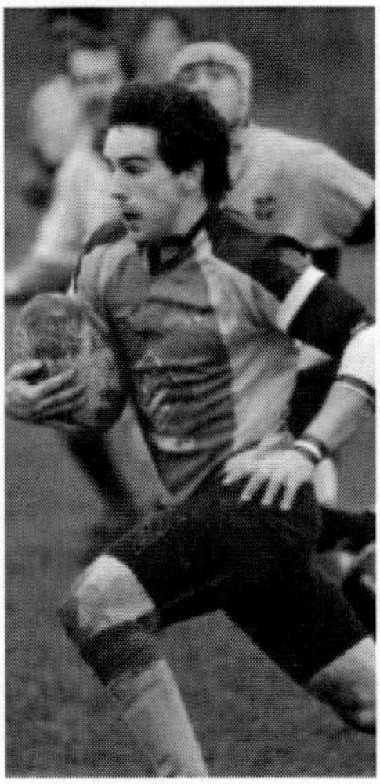

Fig 6.2: Pole vaulting

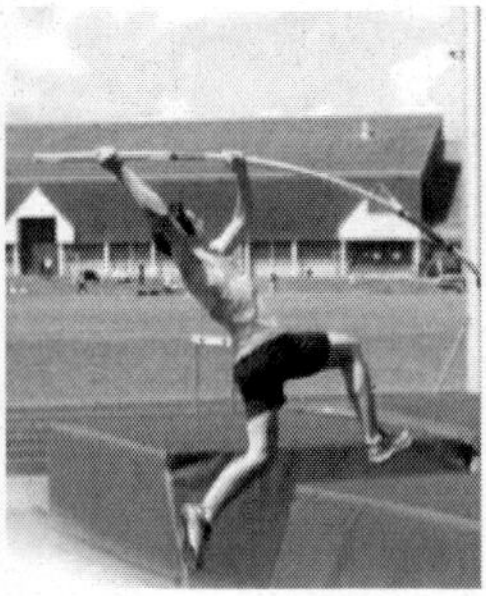

Fig 6.3: Climbing

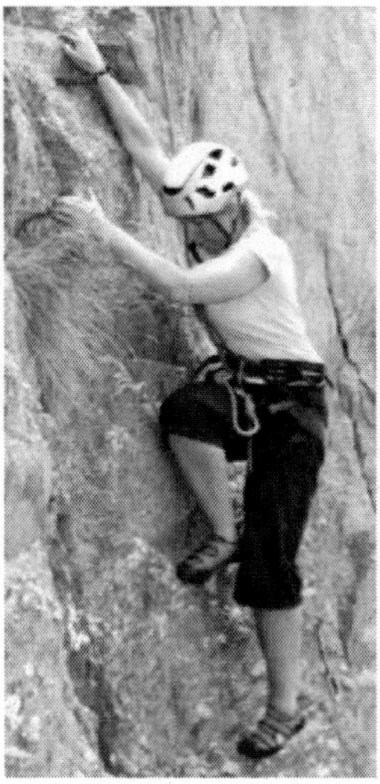

Fig 6.4: Skiing

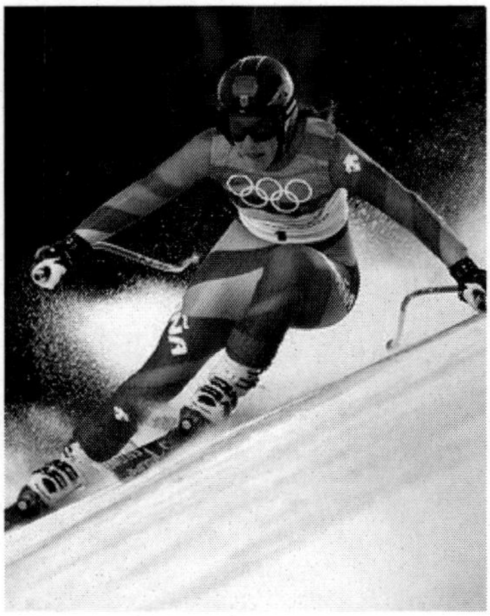

Carolina Ruiz, Vancouver 2010 Olympic Winter Games.

Reproduced with permission from Carolina Ruiz

Fig 6.5: Golf swing

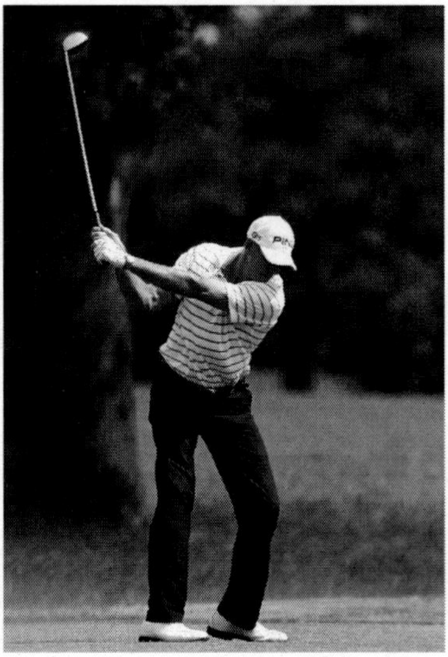

Reproduced with permission from Peter Fowler

When thinking of the anatomical fascial lines involved in sports patterning it is also important to consider other lines. Take a look at the pole vaulter's extended left lateral line, and the closing of his right spiral line, as prepares to make his vault (Figure 6.2). Notice also how the deep front line of the climber's right leg is engaging to give her core extra support as she prepares to extend her hip (Figure 6.3).

If we look at these as common movement patterns, then we can also look at the lines of force that are being engaged. Most sports actions involve connecting the arm to the opposite leg to increase the power. This requires length through the front functional line, shown clearly above in the rugby player's running gait, the pole vaulter's lift off and the climber's pulling pattern (Figures 6.1, 6.2 and 6.3). Ideally these lines should transmit forces evenly throughout the movement patterns, but if there are restrictions in the opposing line then the full range of movement cannot be achieved and the action will have insufficient power. If these excessive strains are allowed to accumulate, or are left untreated, it can result in injury along the line.

As one line shortens, its opposing line lengthens. Think of a bow and arrow. The functional line is much like the bow, which has to have sufficient pre-tension in order to release the arrow to reach its goal, with enough power to achieve both distance and accuracy. As we shorten the line/sling prior to the explosion, we are pre-loading the tension and muscles (the bow) that are required for the 'explosive' movement (the arrow). If we only draw it back a little way, it will not go as far. If we pull it back further it will have the capacity in the movement to control how far or in which direction we want it to go. See Figure 6.4 where the skier contracts her front functional line, extending her opposite right hip as she transfers her body weight to the left leg in preparation for the explosive extension.

The rotational element is also key in most sports patterns. Consider the golf swing (Figure 6.5) where the arm lines, superficial back and spiral lines all need length to enable the golfer to take his swing efficiently.

CHAPTER 7

Sports Pattern Release (SPR) treatment: functional movement patterns

The importance of taking SOAP (subjective, objective, assessment and plan) notes for SPR treatment

Documenting a patient's assessment and treatment are an integral part of the running of any practice for all healthcare providers. Patients expect to spend the first part of any clinical session recording any initial history and being assessed. At subsequent sessions, updates or changes in symptoms and follow up assessments are recorded.

SPR is a remedial treatment that involves recording the positions in which the patient is treated and also the restrictions identified and treated in the tissues. This will change from treatment to treatment and the monitoring of any changes in presentation during a patient's progress is a vital part of the treatment. This recording of data is most necessary for the effective implementation of SPR.

Benefits of SPR treatment

- Increase in range of movement of the entire movement pattern
- Prevention of injury
- Increase in performance
- Increase in strength and subsequently power of that movement pattern

Contra-indications of SPR treatment

Taking a thorough history is of vital importance to any remedial treatment, to help the therapist identify whether or not it is safe to administer SPR. Below is a list of contra-indications and considerations that need to be covered prior to treatment. This list is by no means exhaustive and the consultation will guide the therapist as to the safety and relevance of this type of treatment for the patient in question. If at any point it is unclear as to whether or not the patient should be treated, the therapist should consult the patient's GP or relevant medical professional.

- Acute injury
- Joint instability
- Radicular pain
- Any sensory or motor changes
- Post op (unless it has been cleared by the consultant)
- Osteoarthritis, rheumatoid arthritis or osteoporosis
- Polymyalgia
- Acute muscle spasm
- Pregnancy and post-partum
- Systemic illness

Considerations of SPR treatment

Fibromyalgia: Although it has been found that soft tissue treatment can help patients with fibromyalgia, they often have a much lower tolerance to remedial tissue treatments. If a patient has been diagnosed with fibromyalgia then, although SPR can be used, it must be carried out with the utmost consideration for the patient's pain threshold.

Joint restrictions: During the objective examination, if the patient has joint pain or restriction, this will often need to be looked at first.

The joint should be assessed for injury and, once cleared of inflammation, degenerative conditions, loose bodies, instability or impingements, the joint can be treated with either Mulligan's[16] or Maitland's[17] mobilisations. Both types of mobilisation work well with SPR, if the joint is found to be restricted. In many cases, Mulligan's approach tends to be more complementary to SPR, as it utilises therapist-applied accessory glides with patient-generated active physiological movements. This can be easier to apply during phase two of SPR although, depending on the treatment required, the patient may have to be moved into a different position.

As long as there are no contra-indications and the technique does not cause joint or radicular pain, then there is a great deal which can be done by treating the soft tissue around the associated joint. Often, this alone will have a positive effect on the function of the joint.

Hypermobility: If a patient is hypermobile in one joint, it does not necessarily mean they cannot be treated with SPR. However, a full assessment is necessary to decide whether they are hypermobile in that pattern, or just the individual joint.

If a patient is clinically hypermobile, i.e. has tested positive in the Beighton nine point system (see Table 7.1), then SPR as a treatment would not be beneficial or helpful to that patient. If this is the case, the patient would need to work on their sling strength and additionally would benefit from proprioceptive taping procedures.

Patients under 18: Patients in this category who have not yet finished growing are often still hypermobile. A thorough history-taking and, if necessary, GP consent may be applicable before treating this population.

Table 7.1: Beighton nine point system

Joint	Finding	Points
Left little (fifth) finger	Passive dorsiflexion beyond 90°	1
	Passive dorsiflexion <= 90°	0
Right little (fifth) finger	Passive dorsiflexion beyond 90°	1
	Passive dorsiflexion <= 90°	0
Left thumb	Passive dorsiflexion to the flexor aspect of the forearm	1
	Cannot passively dorsiflex thumb to flexor aspect of the forearm	0
Right thumb	Passive dorsiflexion to the flexor aspect of the forearm	1
	Cannot passively dorsiflex thumb to flexor aspect of the forearm	0
Left elbow	Hyperextends beyond 10°	1
	Extends <= 10	0
Right elbow	Hyperextends beyond 10°	1
	Extends <= 10	0
Left knee	Hyperextends beyond 10°	1
	Extends <= 10	0
Right knee	Hyperextends beyond 10°	1
	Extends <= 10	0
Forward flexion of trunk with knees full extended	Palms and hands can rest flat on the floor	1
	Palms and hands cannot rest flat on the floor	0

The Beighton score was developed to quantify joint laxity and hypermobility. It uses a nine point scoring system: the higher the score the higher the laxity. A patient may be deemed hypermobile if they reach a score of six or higher. The higher the score, the greater the degree of hypermobility. http://www.shoulderdoc.co.uk/article.asp?article=645

SPR works excellently on chronic dysfunction, rather than pain or injury. If a patient has an injury or has had surgery, then this should be treated in a conservative manner and may require written consent from the patient's medical practitioner before commencement of this type of treatment. Once the injury has healed and has regained **normal** pain free movement, SPR treatment can work incredibly well as part of the patient's further rehabilitation and ongoing management for enhanced movement and performance.

Pre-treatment

Prior to treating a patient with SPR it is important to prepare them well for the treatment. It is important that any patient receiving treatment is not dehydrated or hypoglycemic prior to treatment. Advising patients to make sure they have eaten and are hydrated prior to treatment may be applicable.

The treatment should be explained to the patient, in terms of its benefits and the clinical reasoning for selecting it as the treatment of choice.

Additionally, it is advised that the patient is educated as to the method of the technique, explaining that the ranges the limbs will be taken to can sometimes feel a little uncomfortable. Most patients, if they are athletes, will understand and appreciate this. It is best to talk to the patient about diaphragmatic breathing prior to the treatment, making sure they understand its significance and are able to breathe this way.

Post treatment

Many manual therapists will advise their patients to hydrate after treatment, to improve the effects of 'flushing' the body. Although it is courteous to offer a patient a drink, soft tissue manipulation doesn't literally 'flush' or remove 'toxins' but may actually increase the by-products or inflammatory mediators of microscopic injury, particularly during deep tissue work. The delayed onset muscle soreness experienced post treatment is actually a very mild from of myolysis, a breakdown in skeletal muscle tissue. However, although there is some soft tissue work involved in SPR, it is fairly marginal compared to deep tissue manipulation, so any post treatment discomfort of this nature should be minimal.

The patient will feel tired after their treatment. Studies show that prolonged stretching of muscle in the body decreases strength temporarily.[18] It takes time for the brain and central nervous system to process tissue changes and this can make the patient feel quite exhausted.

It is important that the patient is advised **not** to engage in any sporting activity for the 48 hours post treatment. After this they may notice an improvement in their performance, or in the way their body feels.

Practitioner posture

It is not necessary to be strong or powerful to carry out SPR, but a good technique is essential. Taking the patient's limbs into the patterns and having to simultaneously apply pressure in the treatment direction can sometimes be difficult. If not addressed prior to the beginning of a movement, it can leave the therapist in an awkward and posturally compromising position for long periods. This means that the treatment either has to be abandoned, as the therapist is unable to support and treat the limb, or that the therapist injures themself during the treatment.

Firstly, the therapist should ensure that the plinth is the right height and that there is ample space around the treatment table to move the limbs in the full range. Secondly, the therapist should stand as close to the patient as possible to enable adequate support and stability can be applied throughout the treatment. Thirdly, the therapist should adopt either a good lunge stance, or be able to squat effectively whilst keeping the back straight. This will be especially important during the SPR 2 positions, when the more flexible patients' range will require a good stance from the therapist.

The phases of SPR treatment

SPR can be divided into three main phases of treatment:

Diagnostic phase 1: The patient is positioned in a lengthened pattern (see Table 8.1) to identify the areas of tissue that require treatment and the order in which they should be treated.

Treatment phase 2: The area to be treated is slightly shortened, relaxing the tissue.

During this phase, the therapist applies the release, to the primary restriction ('**Key**') in the direction of the pattern being treated. The patient actively moves the limb further into the range, working with the therapist. Where possible the active limb should be supported by the therapist or by a mobilisation belt while the patient moves it (active assisted). The therapist should work with the patient's breathing.

Phase 1 is then repeated to see whether the **Key** needs further treatment, or to find the next restriction in the pattern ('**Link**'). This is repeated until the **Key** and any **Links** have significantly decreased or disappeared and the entire line feels less restricted.

Stretch phase 3: The patient is moved passively into the direction of the pattern the therapist is working in, using diaphragmatic breathing.

Application

In the example below, the patient presents with shoulder stiffness as they begin to reach across their body (as in reaching for a seatbelt).

A useful approach is to begin with the simpler PNF pattern, then progress the patient into a sling or functional line stretch, utilising more of their body to see whether the restrictions are just local (in the PNF pattern), or whether, as they move further into the sports pattern, restrictions are found elsewhere.

SPR can be used to treat a single pattern of gross movement, or several movement ranges. This will depend on the patient and their requirements.

The example below demonstrates how the principles of SPR can be used to treat right shoulder stiffness, during adduction and flexion.

Diagnostic phase 1

The patient is placed supine on the plinth. The right arm is passively moved across the body in the D1 pattern (flexion, adduction, external rotation) (see Figure 5.1). Areas of discomfort or restriction are identified. If there is more than one area then the greatest restriction (**Key**) must be treated first. Let us assume that they report the **Key** in the posterior deltoid.

Treatment phase 2

The patient takes their arm across their body in the D1 pattern, as above. The therapist applies the release along the tissue lines of the posterior deltoid. The **Key** may be a trigger point or a localised pain point or may just feel tight. The treatment is the same. Sustained pressure is applied in the direction of the movement pattern being treated until an ease is felt in the tissue, while the patient reaches further into the pattern as they exhale.

Phase 1, is then repeated to ascertain whether or not there is an improvement in that range, or whether there are further restrictions. If an improvement has been noted, the patient can be passively moved further into that range to identify secondary restrictions (**Links**), which are then treated as above in order of discomfort.

Stretch phase 3

Once an improvement in the range has been noted and the patient is able to move comfortably within the pattern, a passive stretch is applied in this direction. This should be done in conjunction with the patient's diaphragmatic breathing. As they exhale, if a 'give' is felt in the movement, then the limb can be moved further into the D1 pattern.

In certain situations where the dysfunction has been chronic, kinesiotape can be applied in the direction of the movement you are trying to improve, with the limb in the lengthened position. This will help the patient to improve proprioceptive awareness of their renewed tissue length.

References

(16) Mulligan B.R (2006). *Manual Therapy NAGS, SNAGS, MWWMs etc.* 5th ed. New Zealand: Plane View services Ltd.

(17) Prentice, W.E (2004). *Rehabilitation Techniques for Sports Medicine and Athletic Training.* 4th ed. Columbus: McGraw-Hill

(18) Fowles, J.R., et al. (2000). Reduced Strength after passive stretch of Human Plantarflexors. *Journal of Applied Physiology.* 89 (3), 1179-1188

CHAPTER 8

Sports patterns

PARTICULAR SPORTS WILL HAVE patterns that are more specific to them, but for the first few treatments it is advisable to take the patient through all the patterns to help identify and treat the most restricted areas. The theory behind this is because there is a great deal of cross-over in sports patterns across a range of sports.

Subsequent treatments may be more tailored to a specific athlete's particular movement requirements, when restrictive patterns have been identified. It is worth noting here that athletes, on the whole, will have more range in certain patterns then others depending their sport, due to the SAID principle (specific adaptation to imposed demands). This is both specific and necessary.

Fig 8.1: Positioning for a shot

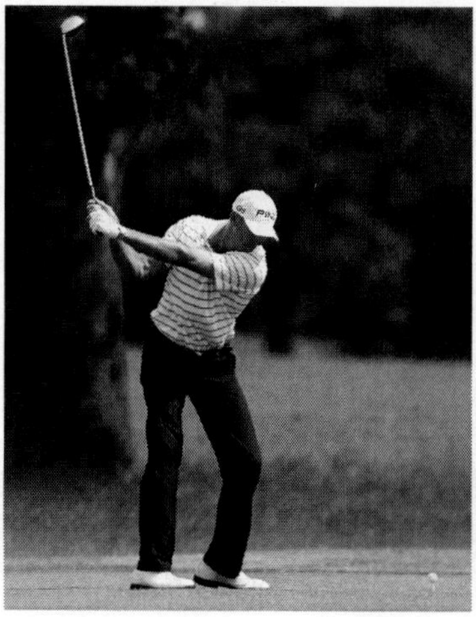

Reproduced with permission from Peter Fowler

Fig 8.2: Following through

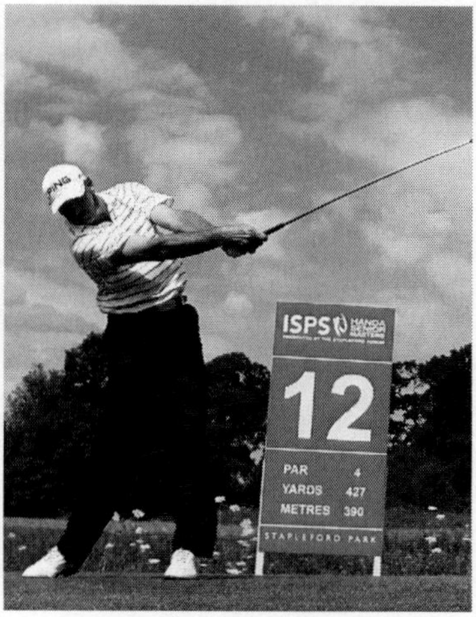

Reproduced with permission from Peter Fowler

Consider the golfer (Figure 8.1). As he positions himself for his shot, he requires length in his back functional line from his left shoulder to his right hip. As he shortens his front functional line, in order to give him the power he needs in his front functional line from his right shoulder to his left hip, he rotates through to take his shot. His right hip to left shoulder lengthens (Figure 8.2) as he follows through, his right shoulder to left hip shortens and his left back functional line contracts lifting the left shoulder and drawing it back and his right shoulder adducts lengthening through his contralateral back functional line.

Other slings are also utilised but, for the purposes of the SPR treatment, we are focusing on the functional lines. This analysis illustrates the utilisation of the functional lines throughout the swing and clarifies the need to assess all SPR positions. By identifying where the athlete is restricted and by releasing those restrictions in the patterns, you can optimise function throughout the necessary range.

In addition, it can transpire that a range where you would expect to find the greatest length, e.g. front functional line from left shoulder to right hip in a striker, can, over time, lead to a restriction in that very range. This is because once muscles and fascia reach full stretch, there is no 'give' left in that range and the joint capsule, with its ligamentous attachments, becomes loaded, often leading to injury. If these inert structures are put under stretch or excessive load, the joint in the range will feel unstable and send neurological messages to the brain to tighten or restrict the soft tissues. This decrease in proprioception can lead to chronic tightness and can be perceived by the brain as its end of range. If this is not addressed, joints in the line of pull can become dysfunctional.

Fig 8.3: Kicking a ball

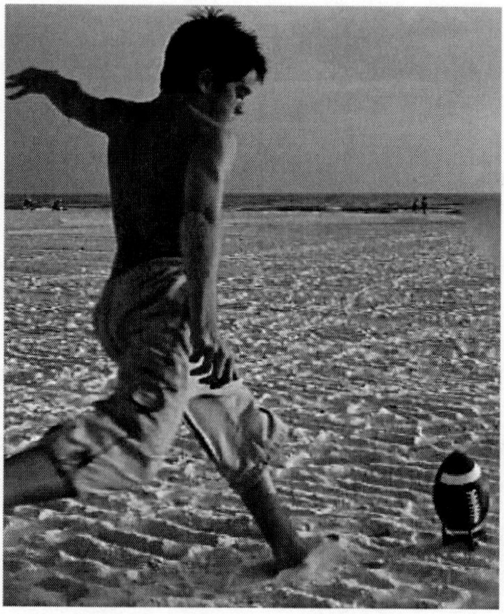

If the right hip is tight in the front functional and deep front lines, as the kicker in Figure 8.3 pre-loads his posterior sling, he will not gain adequate extension through his hip. This will result in more torsion in the back and shoulders during the strike.

The SPR technique helps to promote a balance of mobility and stability in the tissues, helping the athlete to gain optimal function throughout his movement patterns.

Application

Table 8.1 outlines all the SPR ranges. The principles for the application of the technique are described below in some detail using SPR 1 abduction (ABD) as an illustration.

APPLICATION FOR SPR1 ABD

Diagnostic phase 1

1. Place the patient in supine.
2. Take the right hip into full flexion, with knee extended (SLR) to the end of range.
3. From the fully flexed position bring the straight leg into abduction and external rotation to the point where the patient can feel a stretch. At the same time ask them to take their opposite arm into abduction, with external rotation and slight extension (see Figure 8.4). This will be placing the deep front line, the front functional line and the left front arm lines under stretch.
4. Ask the patient to identify the exact point of their greatest source of discomfort, the **Key**.

Treatment phase 2

1. Reduce the abduction/flexion slightly, easing the stretch.
2. Locate the **Key**, which the patient has identified, and ask the patient to inhale and prepare to move actively back into the stretched position.
3. As the patient exhales and actively moves their limb, the therapist applies the release in the same direction, maintaining the pressure until an ease is felt, working with the patient's breathing.
4. The limb is returned to where it was before. It should be more comfortable in that range. The patient is asked to identify the next

most uncomfortable point in the body, the **Link**. Once more the limb is brought back to a comfortable position and the **Link** is worked with a sustained myofascial release in the direction of the movement being worked on. If it is across the midline of the body, the pressure will need to be in the opposite direction. For example, if the **Link** is felt in the pectoralis major, you will need to work in the direction of their arm abduction.

Stretch phase 3

1. Once you have worked on the **Key** and any **Links** in this pattern, you can apply a gentle but slow, progressive, passive stretch in each position, working with the patient's diaphragmatic breathing. Ask them to place their free hand on the base of their ribcage and actively try to move their hand with their breath. Hold the stretch as your patient focuses on their breathing. As they exhale, take the limb a little further into flexion/abduction. Feel the length change in the tissues - do not force the limb. Take your time and work with the patient's breathing. It should now feel like a deep but pain free stretch.

2. If there is any pain, stop. If there is discomfort, it may need more work.

3. Once you are able to take the limb beyond the previous range with no discomfort then you have completed that range.

Table 8.1: The Sports Pattern Release ranges

SPR	Leg	Arm	Fascial line	Postural sling	Figure
SPR1 ABD	Hip ABD/ FL/ER; knee EXT	R arm horizontal ABD/EXT/ ER	Front functional line; front arm lines; deep front line	Anterior oblique	8.4
SPR 2 ABD	Hip horizontal ABD/ER; knee EXT	R arm horizontal ABD/EXT/ ER	Front functional line; front arm lines; deep front line	Anterior oblique	8.5
SPR 3 ABD	Hip ABD/ EXT/ER; knee FL	R arm horizontal ABD/EXT/ ER	Front functional line; front arm line; deep front line	Anterior oblique	8.6
SPR1 ADD	Hip ADD/ FL/IR, knee EXT	R arm ADD/FL/IR	Back functional line; back arm line; lateral line	Posterior oblique	8.7
SPR2 ADD	Hip horizontal ADD/IR; knee EXT	R arm ADD/FL/ IR	Back functional line; back arm line; lateral line	Posterior oblique	8.8
SPR3 ADD	Hip ADD/ IR/; knee EXT	Neck R ROT; L arm FL	Superficial back line/ spiral line	Deep longitu- dinal	8.9

Fig 8.4: SPR 1 abduction/flexion/external rotation

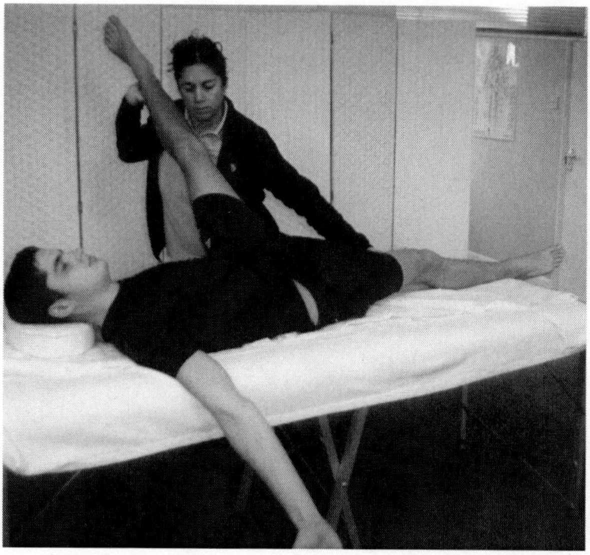

With contra-lateral arm in horizontal abduction/ external rotation

Fig 8.5: SPR 2 horizontal abduction/external rotation

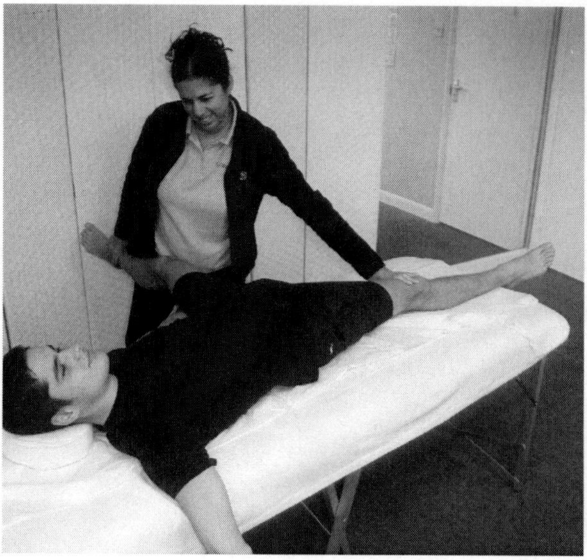

With contra-lateral arm in horizontal abduction/ external rotation

Fig 8.6: SPR 3 abduction/extension/external rotation

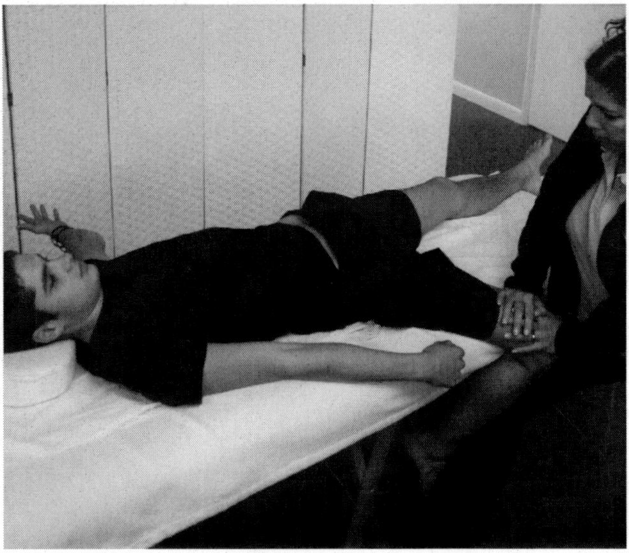

With contra-lateral arm in horizontal abduction/external rotation

Fig 8.7: SPR 1 adduction/flexion/internal rotation

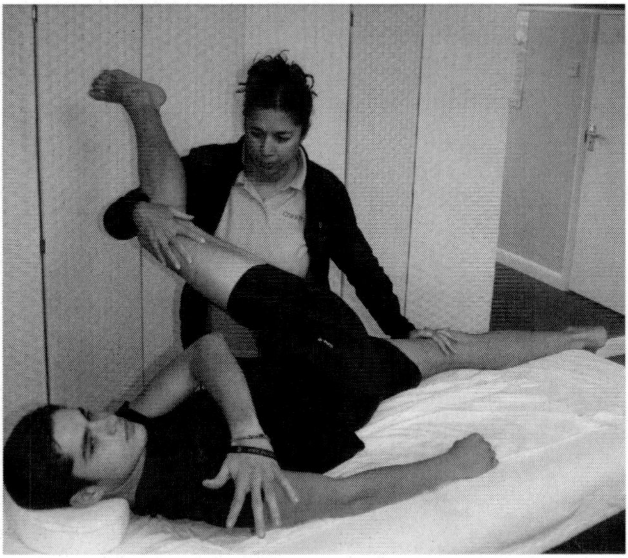

With contra-lateral arm in adduction/flexion/internal rotation

Fig 8.8: SPR 2 horizontal adduction/internal rotation

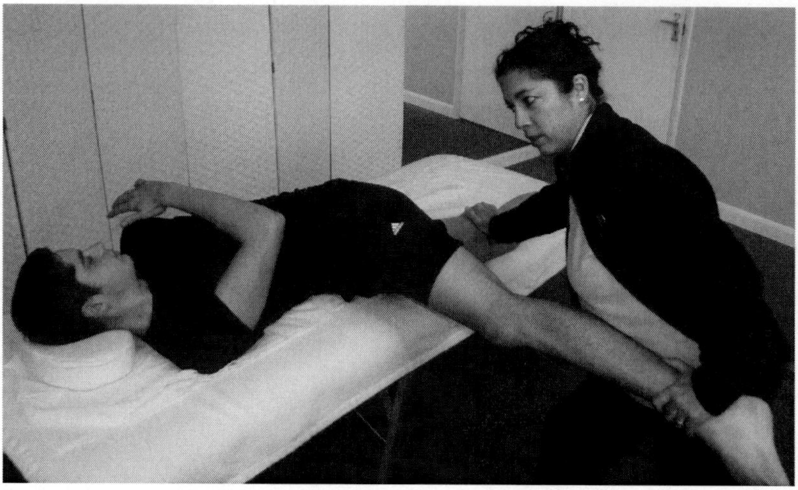

With contra-lateral arm in adduction/flexion/internal rotation

Fig 8.9: SPR 3 adduction/internal rotation

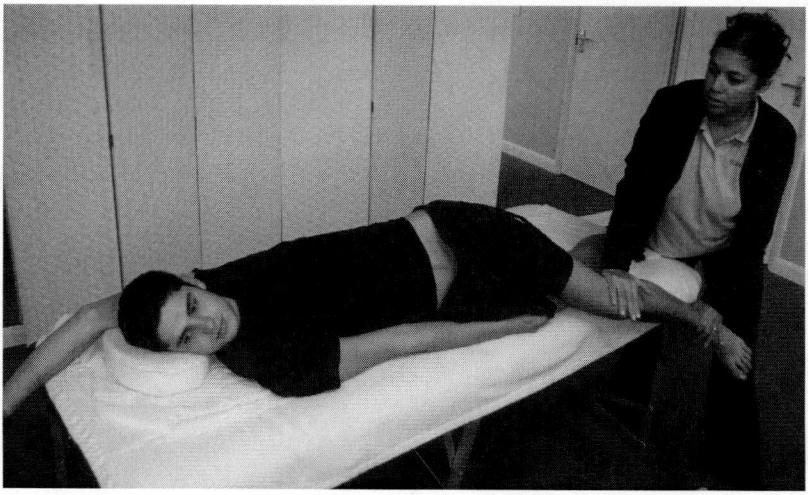

With ipsi-lateral arm in full flexion and neck in rotation

Positions

The patient's lower limb is passively taken into the pattern and the therapist begins to feel the resistance in the tissue as the primary restriction or **Key** is identified. At this point the therapist asks the patient to move their upper body in a particular direction to see if the **Key** intensifies (see Table 8.1). The patient is then asked to move their upper body as far into the direction as they are able, while the therapist holds the lower limb still. For example, if the upper body movement begins with arm adduction they should continue this to thoracic rotation if able to, placing increasing tensile stress through the entire pattern.

In each position the patient will only feel an increase in the restriction by moving the upper body if there are remote restrictions in the pattern. Often the restrictions are found more locally to the lower limb being moved. Sometimes as these are treated, the more remote restrictions (**Links**) can be identified, if they exist. However, this is not always the case.

Remember, every patient is different and will have differences in the way they respond to the treatment.

To summarise Sports Pattern Release

So how does it all work? Why does applying a stretch to movement patterns work so much better than individual muscle stretching?

Well firstly, as discussed at the beginning of this book, muscles do not work individually or in only one direction. Different muscle fibres within the same muscle work in different directions. For example, consider gluteus medius; the anterior fibres work to medially rotate and flex the hip, but the posterior fibres aid in hip extension and external rotation. The same muscle has two completely different sets of fibres that make it work in different directions. To try to apply a stretch to this muscle you would need to apply the stretch in different directions. Most muscles in the body contribute to different movements. This is why to think in terms of movement rather than individual muscles make sense. In this way we can target patterns of restricted motion in our treatment strategies. In addition, the fascia that overlays and interlinks various muscles has lines that follow functional movement, therefore, when we apply a stretch we need to consider this too. As well as this, both fascia and muscle are densely innervated by mechanoreceptors which are responsive to manual pressure. Stimulation of these receptors has been shown to induce a lowering of sympathetic tonus and a change in local tissue viscosity.[19] We are not altering muscle stiffness, but we are stimulating neuromuscular changes in the tissue by convincing the nervous system to allow an increase in range. Using the SPR technique, we are achieving this in functional directions.

Summary of the technique

- The patient is placed in a particular functional pattern, which places the tissues under stretch in that position.
- The restricted areas in this pattern are identified, in order of discomfort.
- The primary area (**Key**) is treated first, in the direction of the movement the therapist is working to improve, working with the patient as they actively move in the same direction.
- The patient is placed back in the same position. If the **Key** is no longer the primary area, or can no longer be identified, the next area of discomfort (**Link**) is treated - again in the direction of the movement pattern.
- The patient should be taken through a passive stretch, in the direction the therapist has been treating for up to 15-30 seconds working with their breathing, once a comfortable range has been reached. This should not take the patient into pain, only minor discomfort.
- The patient can be taken through the full method or worked through areas, which the therapist has identified as the areas most specific to the patient.

- It may take several treatments before a functional change is noticed.
- SPR should be used in conjunction with other treatment modalities for best effects.

References

(19) Schleip, R. (2003). Fascial Plasticity – A new Neurobiological explanation: part 1. *Journal of Bodywork and Movement therapies*. 7 (issue 1)

CHAPTER 9

Yoga for functional and sports performance

EARLIER ON IN THIS BOOK we discussed how the principles of yoga can be applied as an adjunct to Sports Pattern Release (SPR) and how complementary its practice can be to the patient.

Yoga has always embraced the importance of training the body in a sequence of slow sustained stretches, with the holding of a pose not only stretching the opened line but also strengthening the opposing closed line.

For example, if we look at the classic yoga 'dancer' pose, we are stretching the superficial front line, but at the same time we are engaging the superficial back line (see Figure 9.2).

However, the twisting poses are the ones which tend to work the body in the closest way to the SPR technique. They both strengthen and elongate the tissues along the diagonal lines that closely mimic most sporting movements.

In Table 9.1 (overleaf), you will find some of the poses that closely simulate the patterns in particular sports. Encouraging patients to engage in this type of exercise will enhance SPR work with them and will also enhance their performance as an athlete.

Table 9.1 is an exercise compendium of yoga-pose examples that can be used to guide patients to maintain the changes in their body, based on yoga stretches for particular fascial lines, relative to the most common sports discussed earlier in the book.

Table 9.1

Sport	Lengthened fascial lines/ slings	Sports pattern lengthened	Yoga pose	Figure
Soccer: kick-follow through	Back functional/ posterior sling	SPR1 ADD	Twisting triangle	9.1
Soccer: kick aim	Front functional/ anterior sling	SP3 ABD	Dancer	9.2
Tennis: serve	Front functional/ anterior sling	SPR3 ABD	Sun warrior/ Swan	9.3 9.4
	Lateral Line (Deep front line/ lateral and anterior sling	SPR2 ABD	Half moon/ Gate pose/ Triangle	9.5 9.6 9.7
Tennis: underhand	Back & front functional/ posterior & anterior sling	SPR1 ADD	Lunge twist	9.8
Golf: swing	Back functional/ posterior sling	SPR1 ADD	Prayer twist	9.9
Running	Superficial front line/ anterior sling	SPR3 ABD SPR2 ADD	Warrior 1/ Low lunge twist	9.10 9.11
Pole vault	Back & front functional/ posterior & anterior sling	SPR1 ADD SPR3 ABD	Lunge twist	9.8
Skiing	Back functional/ posterior sling	SPR1 ADD	Prayer twist	9.9

The deep front line is known as the 'up' line in yoga. It is specific to most movement patterns and can be considered the key element to strengthening the core. Commands from yoga teachers involving the teaching of exercises to activate this line are about lifting and engaging.

For example, "pick up the inner arch of the foot", "lift the inner thighs", "pull up through the pelvic floor", "lift the patellae" and "find length in your spine and grow tall through the crown of the head" - all of these cues are associated with axial core support and the deep front line.

Looking at the yoga poses, we can see how many of them lengthen several lines concurrently and also strengthen opposing lines.

The triangle pose (Figure 9.7) lengthens the deep front line, the lateral and the front functional lines at the same time. In addition, it both stretches and strengthens the deep front line and the lateral lines simultaneously (as one side is worked, the other can lengthen and vice versa).

Furthermore, many of the twisting poses will lengthen the anterior and posterior aspects of the body during the same pose. For example, in the lunge twist (Figure 9.8), although the model's anterior sling/functional line is the line predominantly being stretched from her left hip through to right shoulder, her posterior sling/functional line is also being lengthened from her right hip to left shoulder.

Utilising specific yoga practice along with other relevant rehabilitation exercises, which have been prescriptively selected by the therapist, will enhance the SPR treatment, helping the patient to achieve greater results and maintain balance throughout their body.

NB: It is advisable to work with a qualified yoga instructor, or sports/ physical therapist who has experience in this field, to learn the safest and most effective execution of this type of exercise.

Fig 9.1: Twisting triangle

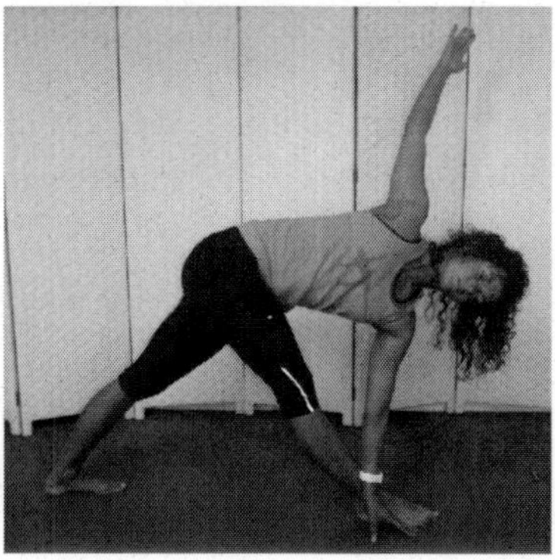

Fig 9.2: Dancer

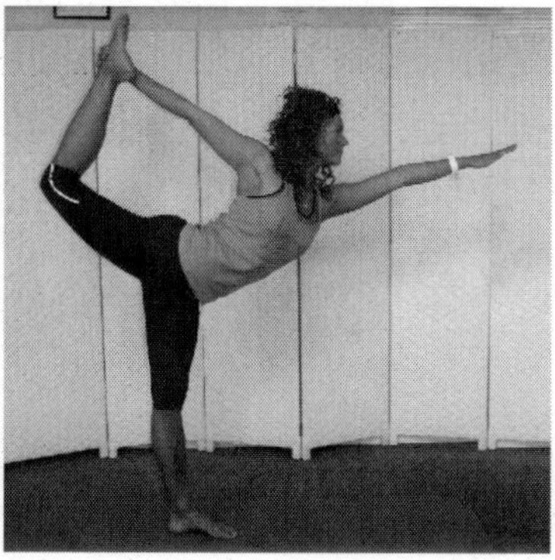

Fig 9.3: Sun warrior

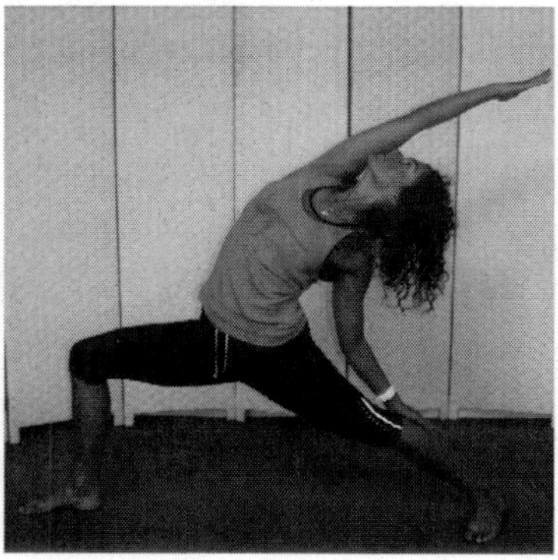

Fig 9.4: Swan

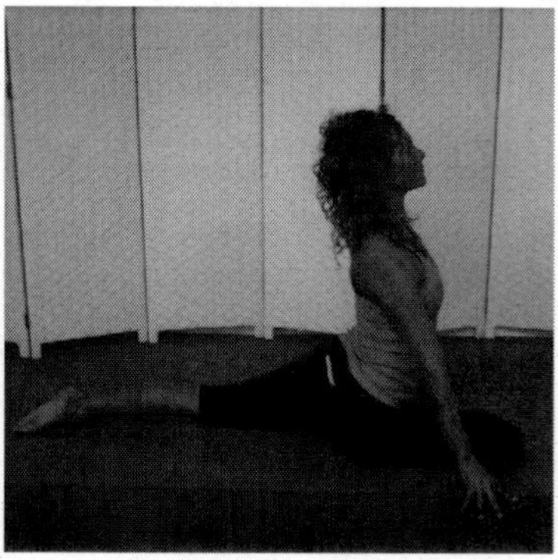

Fig 9.5: Half moon

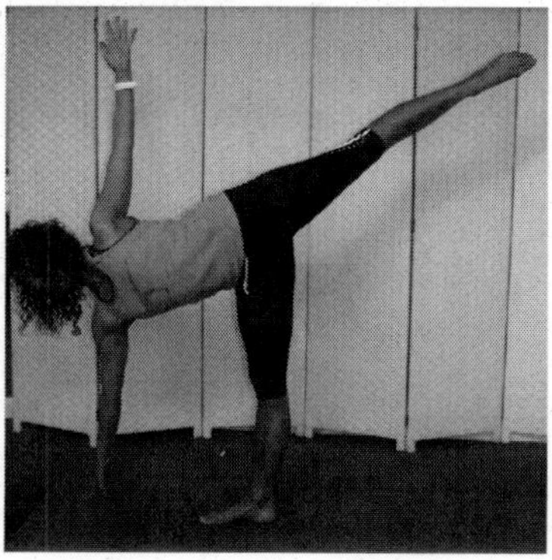

Fig 9.6: Gate

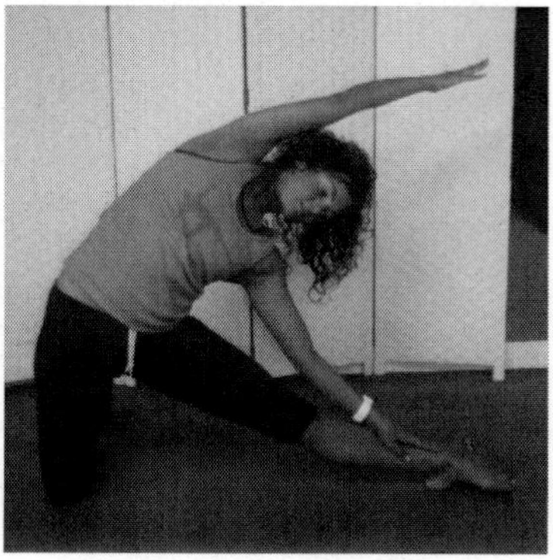

Fig 9.7: Triangle

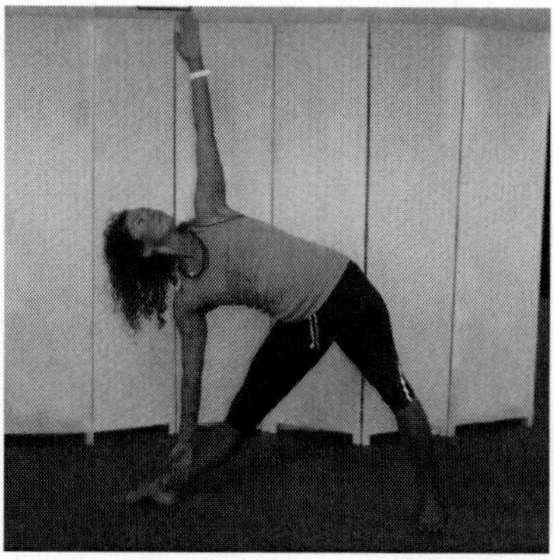

Fig 9.8: Lunge twist

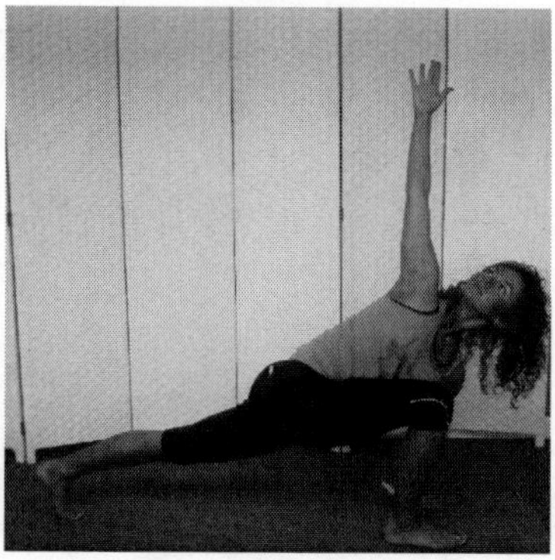

Fig 9.9: Prayer twist

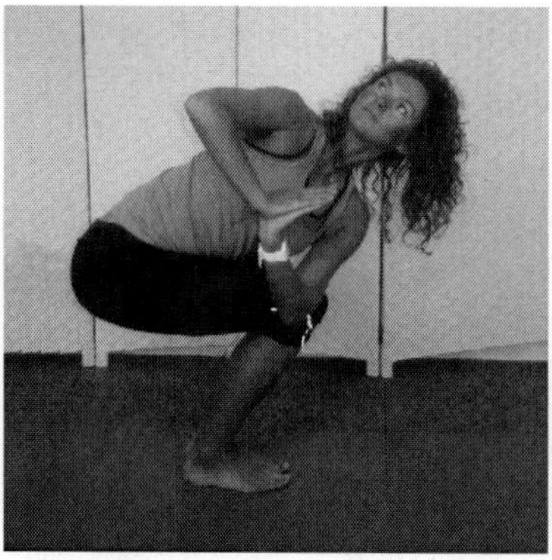

Fig 9.10: Warrior 1

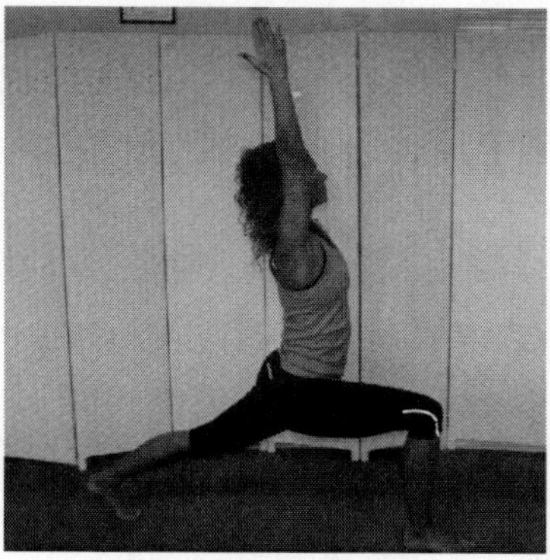

Fig 9.11: Low lunge twist

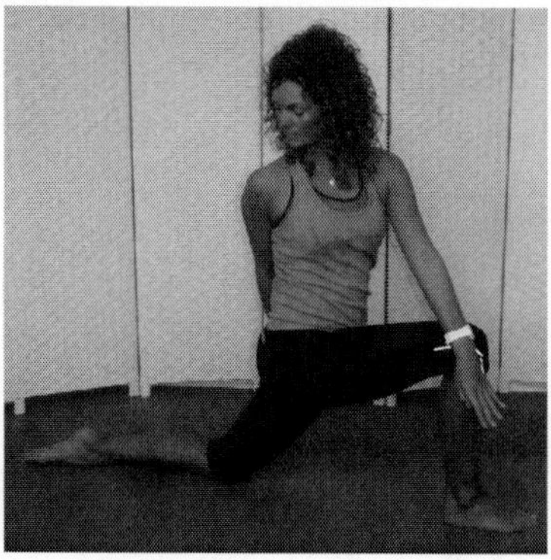

CHAPTER 10

Sports Pattern Release (SPR) for common disfunctions

ALTHOUGH FOR GENERAL SPORTS pattern lengthening it works well to use the whole SPR model, for specific dysfunctions, particular pattern release becomes more appropriate later on in the patient's treatment programme. Placing the patient in the SPR pattern will identify the **Key** restrictions, enabling the therapist to work through them, releasing the pattern in order of restriction. Once the restrictions have been treated, the patient can be advised on their rehabilitation. This will be based on strengthening the weakened pattern or sling and maintaining the length in the shortened or restricted pattern.

The more experience the therapist has of both identifying specific dysfunction and of working with SPR, the easier it becomes to select a treatment regime for the dysfunction. The list below gives a few examples of SPR techniques that can be applied to some common presentations. The list is by no means exhaustive and it should be noted that, if other factors also contribute to the patient's dysfunction, then other patterns may be applied instead of or as well as those listed. Additionally, as previously stated, it may be necessary to treat conservatively prior to or as well as using SPR, if the dysfunction is associated with acute injury or if there is an underlying cause.

Table 10.1: List of treatment patterns for common dysfunctions

Dysfunction	Presentation	SPR	Sling targeted	Sling rehab focus
Anteriorly translated gleno-humeral joint	Shoulder pain particularly on full flexion	SPR 3 ABD	Anterior oblique	Posterior oblique
Sacro-iliac or pelvic rotation	Hip pain/ stiffness on load bearing forward flexion	SPR 3 ADD	Deep longi-tudinal	Anterior oblique
Delayed or inhibited glut max firing	Low back pain	SPR 1 ADD	Posterior oblique	Posterior oblique*
Groin strain or osteitis pubis	Overactive adductors; restricted ribs and diaphragm	SPR 3 ABD	Anterior oblique	
Patella femoral syndrome	Overactive TFL; inhibited glut med	SPR 3 ABD	Anterior oblique	Lateral
Ankle sprains (chronic; repetitive)	Inhibited glut med, and ipsilateral adductors	SPR 3 ADD	Deep longi-tudinal	Lateral
Achilles pain (chronic; no local, acute inflam-mation)	Overactive lateral gastrocnemius	SPR 2 ADD	Posterior oblique	Ipsi-lateral deep longi-tudinal

* NB: Often the pattern, or at least parts of it, that needs to be released will also form all or part of the sling or pattern that needs to be strengthened. This is because the restrictions in that pattern inhibit the

correct firing of other muscles in the sling. Once these restrictions are treated, then the sling can be strengthened as a whole without the overactive structures dominating the pattern. This encourages efficiency throughout the entire pattern.

INDEX

Made in United States
North Haven, CT
04 November 2026

21771222R00053